AROMA BUMP

The Belly Bible for Aromatherapy in Pregnancy

LISA HEENEY

authorHOUSE®

AuthorHouse™ UK
1663 Liberty Drive
Bloomington, IN 47403 USA
www.authorhouse.co.uk
Phone: 0800.197.4150

Published by AuthorHouse 11/07/2016

ISBN: 978-1-5246-6263-9 (sc)
ISBN: 978-1-5246-6264-6 (hc)
ISBN: 978-1-5246-6262-2 (e)

Print information available on the last page.

To my lovely husband John, who says I'm a great one for the ideas.

Contents

Preface

I WAS FIRST introduced to essential oils in the year 2000 when I went for some reflexology treatments from a wonderful lady called Nancy Hynes, who was also an aromatherapist. I loved how I felt after receiving Nancy's treatments, and she would often send me home with a little bottle filled with the remainder of the essential oil blend she had been using. The blends smelled gorgeous, and I found them to be extremely restorative and comforting. My only brother, Kevin, had died suddenly at the beginning of that same year and I was in a very low mental space as a result. Little did the lovely Nancy know that she would become a key influencer in what would later become an integral part of my life, and work.

In 2001 after completing my reflexology diploma (once again as a direct result of Nancy's influence), I immediately started a diploma in Holistic Aromatherapy in the prestigious Tisserand Institute of Aromatherapy in London. Prior to the diploma starting, I had taken part in a magazine competition to win a scholarship for the aromatherapy diploma in Tisserand, which as fate would have it, a nun from my secondary school, Sr. Patricia, had brought to my attention (Thank you Sr. Patricia!). It turns out that I came second, so no scholarship was won. However, I felt so strongly about learning more about essential oils that I proceeded to apply for the course anyway and travelled from Dublin to London on a monthly basis for two years to attend the weekend seminars.

Having qualified as an aromatherapist, and despite not yet having children of my own at that time, I had a keen interest in working with pregnancy.

I found it amazing and something to be celebrated and supported. I was building up a loyal clientele working as The Pregnancy Reflexologist, and I was also offering aromatherapy pregnancy massage. Many clients had begun to ask me for aromatherapy advice, in terms of which essential oils to use at home to help with certain discomforts they were experiencing.

In 2008 I was pregnant with my first child and I referred often to my list of essential oils with the aim of easing the normal aches and pains of pregnancy life. I used aromatherapy blends in the bath, in body oils, facial creams and in my trusty oil burner around my home, and I found that they helped me in so many aspects. Baby number 2 came along in 2010, and once again the essential oils played an important role in keeping me happy and healthy in my pregnancy.

Somewhere between having my second baby and being pregnant with my third, the idea about writing an aromatherapy book for pregnancy started to germinate in my head. I felt that essential oils had helped me so much in my own pregnancies that I would like to share that information with other pregnant women, so that they too could experience the benefits. I saw too on social media that there were many discussions regarding the use of essential oils in pregnancy and labour. I realised that there were many questions, and unfortunately, some of the answers, even though they may have been given in good faith, were not always correct, or safe. Here, I felt that I could put my knowledge of both aromatherapy and pregnancy to good use by compiling helpful information that women could use with confidence that would support them in their pregnancies, in labour and post-partum.

And so the plan to write AromaBump was put into action. Overall, the whole process has taken me four years to complete – that's what having three children in the space of four and a half years did for my work productivity levels! Anyway, it is said that good things are worth the wait… so here it is, and it comes down to this: My one wish for you is that you enjoy using this book and the aromatherapy blends that it contains, and that you and your baby carry wellness, both in your pregnancy, and once baby is born, wherever you go.

Acknowledgements

A SPECIAL THANKS for the love and support given to me by my wonderful husband, John, my family, my lovely wee mummy, and my fantastic parents-in-law, who are always there to dig me out of a hole, be it with child-minding, a flat tyre, or a leaky roof.

I would like to acknowledge the input of my best friend called Helen, whose support at the beginning of this project enabled me to get the ball rolling. I would also like to acknowledge the encouragement and direction given to me by my friend, coach and cheerleader, Cara, without whose help, I fear, this book would have taken even longer to complete!

I would also like to thank the very talented Bridget from Bammedia for designing my book cover – she has been able to make superbly tangible that which was previously only in my head.

And finally, a special mention to my beautiful ladies who have come to me for reflexology and aromatherapy treatments - thank you for letting me share even a little part of your pregnancy experience, and for everything that I learn from you on a daily basis.

Thank you, and much love to you all!

Introduction

PREGNANCY IS A very exciting time and if it's your first time being pregnant, then absolutely everything is new. I know the feeling of wanting to know everything about everything, and how, suddenly, you feel that you want to consume all that is pregnancy related. One thing is for sure, being positively supported, and building your tool kit to feel happy and well in your pregnancy is fundamental. There are many ways to do this such as taking care of your physical health through proper nutrition, exercise and rest; and mentally, through the fabulous brain training for birth programmes that are currently available. Aromatherapy is another fantastic way of helping to look after your physical and mental health in pregnancy and this book, AromaBump, addresses how the proper use of essential oils can enhance a woman's pregnancy throughout the three trimesters, in labour, as well as in the post-partum period.

In this book, you will find a practical guide to using, and benefiting from aromatherapy for pregnancy in an educated and safe way. You will be given details on 24 different essential oils and have access to dozens of exclusive aromatherapy blends for you to make and use at home. We will address 27 separate discomforts that are common in pregnancy and show how they can be improved using aromatherapy. Furthermore, we will also take a closer look at how your pregnancy skin can change, and how to treat skin conditions differently now that you are pregnant. Finally, we will learn how to ease any post-partum and breast-feeding discomforts that you may experience, using essential oils. I share with you how to blend essential oils correctly so that you are using the right amount, and profile beneficial carrier oils that you can use in your blends.

There is no doubt that the word, 'aromatherapy' has become very popular over the last 20 years, with it appearing on many cosmetic labels, air-fresheners, foodstuffs, and even laundry products. However, aromatherapy is more than just pretty smells, and the widespread use of the term has perhaps distracted from the real focus of how we can use plant essences in a properly beneficial and therapeutic way.

In its true form, aromatherapy is the use of essential oils to evoke a beneficial action on a person's well-being, by improving their physical, mental, and emotional state. This means that by using essential oils, there are many aspects of our being that we can affect positively.

But what are essential oils really? Perhaps, paradoxically, they are not really an oil. However, they are the fragrant essences that can be extracted from all types of plants normally by the use of steam distillation, cold pressing or CO_2 extraction, for their healing properties. They are extremely potent, and a little goes a long way. Being completely natural substances, they are not to be confused with synthetically formulated fragrance oils which offer neither therapeutic nor healing benefits.

Essential oils can be used to enhance well-being in a number of ways and can be used in a variety of manners. AromaBump gives details of the most common means of effective application, and exposure to them, which are:

- Massage - A specific blend of essential oils is created to address presenting issues or conditions and diluted in a vegetable carrier oil. This is then applied to the skin using therapeutic massage techniques.
- Bath - A particular blend of essential oils is created and diluted in a vegetable carrier oil and added to a warm bath.
- Inhalation (through vaporisation, or diffusion) - Specific essential oils can be added to the likes of a facial sauna and can then be inhaled directly by placing the face within breathing

distance of the steam source*. If you have an oil burner, 3 or 4 drops of essential oils can be added to the water, which then evaporate around your room. (*Use caution with your steam vaporiser so that you do not have your face overly close to the steam source to avoid burning yourself).

- Dermal application - Essential oils can be incorporated into the formulation of face and body products and then applied onto the skin in creams, lotions, balms or gels.

As a professional aromatherapist who specialises in pregnancy treatments, and as a mother of three children, the information that I am sharing with you in this book is the sort of information that I use when working with my clients, which I also found beneficial as I journeyed through my own pregnancies. AromaBump reveals little gems of aromatherapy and essential oil knowledge that you can put to use on a daily basis to support you in your pregnancy, in an effective, but always safe way. I hope you enjoy using this book, and whether you are someone who already uses essential oils and is familiar with their benefits, or someone who is knocking on aromatherapy's door for the first time, I wish you a beautifully fragrant and happy pregnancy!

For bonus information and additional supporting videos, please visit my website www.AromaBump.com

Disclaimer

THE INFORMATION PROVIDED in this book is all in accordance with the teachings of professional aromatherapy practice, and current essential oil research. However, it is not intended to replace medical advice, and you are kindly reminded to consult with your primary health care provider regarding your health and that of your baby in pregnancy. Furthermore, please note that the information contained in this book is for personal use and does not qualify the user to employ it in a professional aromatherapy context.

CHAPTER 1

Aromatherapy in Pregnancy

AROMATHERAPY IN PREGNANCY can be wonderfully rewarding, positively affecting the mother-to-be, and her developing baby, in a number of ways. Essential oils are naturally occurring substances, however, this does not mean that they can be used excessively, or without caution. In fact, quite the opposite as it is vital to be aware of their respective precautions and contra-indications, and to use essential oils safely and appropriately. This book lists 24 essential oils that can be used in pregnancy and childbirth. There are also sections on dilutions, blends, and recipe suggestions for you to try out at home.

In pregnancy, it is extremely important to be aware of what you are putting ON your body just as much as it is about what you are putting IN your body, as "Most chemicals which are applied to the skin are absorbed to some degree. However, the skin is still an important protective barrier, limiting the rate at which potentially toxic substances gain entry into the body."[1] It is sometimes easy to forget that our skin is the body's largest organ, and it has many functions including:

- Regulation of body temperature - the skin allows the body to lose heat by increasing blood flow close to the skin, helping internal heat to escape. It also facilitates the sweat glands in their functioning, providing the platform from which they allow

[1] Tisserand & Balacs, "Essential Oil Safety 1st ed." 1995, p27

1

sweat to escape from the body, thereby helping it to cool down. The skin also helps the body to heat up by using the shivering mechanism, and also by constricting blood flow at its surface, keeping heat internally where it is needed.

- Protective barrier - It protects internal tissues from the outside environment, and prevents outside invaders from gaining entry. It prevents excess evaporation of water from inside our body and also prevents water from entering the body through the skin when for example, we take a bath or go swimming.
- Facilitates the sense of touch - the skin contains sensory nerve endings that allows us to feel touch, and also the sensation of heat and cold.
- Absorption and excretion - the skin enables the body to lose water and heat by sweating, and also allows certain substances to be absorbed into the body, like fat-soluble vitamins (A, D, E & K). Certain toxic substances can also be absorbed into the body via the skin, as well as constituents of certain heavy metals.[2]
- Synthesis of Vitamin D - the skin houses molecules that upon activation by UV light can be converted by the liver and kidneys into a usable form of Vitamin D.

As you can imagine, the skin's functions become even more important in pregnancy as our body often needs to sweat more and get rid of extra waste products more efficiently. It also needs to protect not only us from external invaders, or threats, but also our developing baby. We need to avoid exposure to unnecessary toxins so as to keep baby safe and also, in order to support both our own and our baby's musculo-skeletal health, we must be able to synthesize vitamin D as effectively as possible.

Natural vs. Synthetic

There are many benefits to using natural compounds over their synthetic counterparts given that they are substances that the body can work

---

[2] Tortora/Grabowski, "Principles of Anatomy and Physiology 9th ed." 2000, p151

with, and can be metabolised more readily. They are made up of many chemical constituents, some of which have fat soluble elements enabling them to permeate the skin, and carry the true essence and energy of the plant into the bloodstream and brain. They trigger real and often rapid responses in the body, like lowering the heart rate, increasing endorphin production, or reducing the inflammatory response, and can be metabolized more readily by the liver and kidneys when no longer needed. Research has shown that essential oils are healing in nature, and therefore can display many benefits for pregnant women through their antibacterial, antiviral, antimicrobial, sleep-inducing, pain-relieving, and excess fluid-reducing properties.

Synthetic fragrance compounds, on the other hand, are manufactured, lifeless substances, which are designed to have an attractive smell for use in industries such as mainstream cosmetics, personal care, and the food industry. They offer no therapeutic value. Furthermore, for many of these synthetic compounds, their chemical composition has rendered them toxic both to the human body and to our environment, increasing the incidence of the likes of allergies, sensitisation, hormone disruption, organ toxicity, asthma, eczema, psoriasis and dermatitis. According to leading toxicologist Dr. Samuel Epstein, "the synthetic nature of most perfumes and fragrances may pose a toxic hazard through avoidable carcinogenic exposure."[3]

During pregnancy, the placenta is the site of exchange between the woman and her baby. One of the primary functions of the placenta is to facilitate the exchange of oxygen and nutrients from the mother's blood into the foetal blood, while carbon dioxide and waste products diffuse from the foetal blood into the maternal blood. According to Tortora and Grabowski, "Almost all drugs, including alcohol and many other substances that can cause birth defects, pass freely through the placenta."[4] Unfortunately, many of these 'other substances' that can cross

---

[3] "Unreasonable Risk – How to avoid cancer from cosmetics and personal care products" by Samuel S. Epstein, M.D., 2001
[4] "Principles of Anatomy and Physiology – 9th ed." by Gerard J. Tortora, Sandra Reynolds Grabowski, 2000

the placental barrier include the aforementioned synthetic fragrance compounds due to the makeup of their molecules.

Synthetic compounds exert stress on a woman's body systems, making her organs work harder to break them down and eliminate them from her body. This diverts energy to these processes; energy that could be directed towards keeping her own immune system strong and to sharing her resources with her baby, but are instead being used up in less important processes. It's like when you are distracted from your main focus - you have less energy to give to what should be the most important thing for you to concentrate on when you have distractions elsewhere. They create responses from the immune system as many of the chemical constituents are considered foreign bodies, to be eliminated.

If synthetic compounds pass from the mother's blood to that of her baby, consequently the baby's organs are subjected to stress from a very early age as they try to either assimilate these compounds into the body or break them down so that they can be excreted. Again, all of this diverts energy away from the most important functions like growth and proper development.

However, as opposed to the potential risks of using synthetic substances, just because a substance is naturally occurring, does not mean that it should be used without caution or proper education. Natural does not automatically mean safe and we will look at this further in the next chapter when we find out how to blend essential oils safely.

CHAPTER 2

It's all in the mix — Proper Blending and Dilution of Essential Oils in Pregnancy

IN ORDER TO use essential oils in a way that is safe and therapeutic for you and your developing baby, they must be diluted in a carrier oil before applying them in any way to your skin.

Unfortunately there is much misinformation currently being circulated by non-aromatherapists which recommends the undiluted or neat use of essential oils on the skin, and even advocates ingesting the essential oils by drinking them in water or a carrier oil like olive oil. This information is not only incorrect, but also irresponsible and highly unsafe. **Please always dilute your essential oils properly in an appropriate carrier oil before using them directly on your skin, or that of your children, and do not drink them.** Details of carrier oils are given in Chapter 4.

The safe dilution for essential oil usage for dermal application in pregnancy is, in a clinical setting, between 1% and 4%. For personal use in a home setting, we are going to use a maximum of a 1% dilution. So, let's work backwards so that we can get a better understanding of how potent essential oils really are. If you use an essential oil straight out of its bottle, that is referred to as being neat, or at 100% strength. When undiluted like this, you can use the essential oil in a diffuser or oil burner, and it will happily evaporate through the air in your room. However, if you plan on using your essential oils on your skin, in a bath, or as part of a cosmetic product, you need to dilute the strength by combining them with a carrier oil like sweet almond, grapeseed, jojoba, or any of the liquid oils referred to in Chapter 4 - Vegetable Oils and Plant Butters, or in another base product like a cream or a gel.

If we want a 1% dilution, we can use 99% of carrier oil, and 1% of essential oil content. This means that whether you are using one essential oil in your blend, or three or four, the total essential oil content should always be 1% of the mix. One drop of essential oil measures on average 0.04ml, (depending on your dropper bottle, some drops measure as little as 0.03ml and others as much as 0.05ml) and this is a good number to remember when you are making up your blends.

If we use a 100ml bottle for our blend, we can add 99ml of carrier oil and 1ml of essential oil(s). This means that we can use 25 drops, in total, of essential oil in a 100ml bottle.

You may be thinking that 1% dilution sounds like a very small amount and would only form a very weak solution. However, with a 1% dilution, you can still be assured that your blend of essential oils is of a therapeutic level, and even more importantly, that it is safe for you and your developing baby. If 1% dilution is still powerful enough to encourage a positive reaction in the body and brain, can you imagine the body's reaction to undiluted essential oil usage? With aromatherapy, the phrase 'less is more' applies more often than not, and higher essential oil dilution does not necessarily mean a better or increased therapeutic reaction.

Quick Dilution Guide to Create a 1% blend

Volume of Carrier Oil/Base Product	Total Drops of Essential Oil
100ml	25
50ml	13
30ml	8
10ml	3

What makes a good blend?

So, what makes a good blend? When considering this, we have to remember that this book has not been written to explain the in-depth scientific background of essential oils, or to delve into the specific chemical profiling of each oil. Therefore, we are going to blend according to the most prominent therapeutic characteristic of the essential oil in question, and its fragrance. In the individual profiles of the essential oils in Chapter 3, you will notice a column entitled 'Blending Note', and top, middle or base being listed per oil. A top note essential oil will evaporate rapidly with its fragrance all but disappearing after a relatively short time. Examples of top note essential oils are mostly citrus oils like lemon, bergamot and grapefruit. A blend of purely top note essential oils would smell very light and have no substantial fragrant depth to it. This would be fine in a diffuser or vaporiser, and there's absolutely nothing wrong with a blend like this, only that there would be little differentiation in its therapeutic value as all of these oils have similar actions.

It is more beneficial in terms of fragrance and general blend aesthetics to use a more balanced mixture that includes top, middle, and base note essential oils. Furthermore, as a general rule of thumb, there would be more drops of a top note essential oil in a blend compared to a base note essential oil. If top, middle, and base note essential oils were used in equal quantities, the less volatile base notes would easily overpower the top ones, lending itself to a very heavy, strong-smelling blend. If you have a good balance of essential oils in your mix, it will result in an appealing fragrance that can develop even more beautifully as you use it. If you are using the blend in a massage or in the bath, you will be first aware of the lighter top and middle notes, and then the depth and maturity of the blend become apparent as the heavier, base note essential oils begin to make their presence felt.

	TOP	MIDDLE	BASE
CITRUS	Bergamot Grapefruit Lemon Mandarin Sweet Orange		
EARTHY		Patchouli	Vetiver
FLORAL	Clary Sage	Geranium Lavender Neroli Roman Chamomile	Rose Ylang Ylang
MEDICINAL	Fragonia	Eucalyptus	Peppermint
SPICEY		Cardamom Cubeb Ginger	
WOODY	Cypress Rosewood	Frankincense	Atlas Cedarwood Sandalwood

Visual Overview of General Characteristics of Essential Oils

Different carrier oils affect the rate of absorption of your essential oils as well. Without a carrier oil, an essential oil will rapidly cross the skin's semi-permeable barrier, and there will quickly be evidence of it in the bloodstream. Essential oils help to draw carrier oils downwards into the lower levels of the skin, and not the other way round. There will be a moderate rate of absorption if you are using a carrier oil like grapeseed or sweet almond oil. However, there will be a much slower rate of overall absorption if you choose to use a carrier oil like jojoba or olive oil as their molecules are bigger and need longer to be assimilated into the body via the fatty layers of the skin. However, if your essential oils are blended in a gel, then there will be a very rapid absorption rate.

When mixing your oils, you can take into consideration what function you would like them to accomplish, how you are going to use the blend (vaporisation, dermal application with a skin product, a massage oil or bath oil), and where on your body you would like to use the blend. Thicker areas of skin will allow for a slower absorption rate (like the base of your heel), and thinner skin such as you would find on the inside of your arms or thighs, or on the face are conducive to a quicker rate of absorption into the body.

For example, rosehip or apricot kernel carrier oils are perfect for use on the face as they are light and rapidly absorbed, whereas carrier oils with a slower rate of absorption, like olive oil or jojoba oil are good to use as part of a blend for a leave-on product, so as to allow proper, long-term exposure to the essential oils blended therein.

NOTE ABOUT STORAGE:

Essential oils are subject to oxidation because they can 'go off', or lose some of their therapeutic benefits. Oxidation in some instances, like lemon, or sweet orange, can also cause some skin reactions or irritation. To avoid this, you must first ensure that you are buying your essential oils from a reputable aromatherapy company, and only buy them if the label says, "Pure Essential Oil", and are packaged in a dark glass bottle like amber (which is best) or dark blue. If possible, keep your essential oils in the fridge as they will last longer. For example, if you have a citrus oil like lemon or grapefruit, it will be good for about 6 months if you store it at room temperature. However, it will last for about 1 year if it is kept in the fridge. Other essential oils if stored at room temperature will last for about 1 year, but at least 2 years if stored in the fridge. Moreover, some essential oils, like patchouli, actually improve with age, certainly in terms of fragrance. There is an aged version of patchouli essential oil that is held in high regard due to its beautiful fragrance, and is labelled, 'Old Patchouli'.

If you are unable to keep your essential oils in a fridge, at least make sure they are away from direct sources of heat and light. (Bathroom or kitchen windowsills are often the main offenders.) Always remember to replace the cap tightly, and immediately after each use of your oil.

In many instances, it is also better for carrier oils to be kept in the fridge, as they too, can easily turn rancid, especially ones that have a high content of polyunsaturates. It may be easier to notice if a carrier oil rather than an essential oil has gone off because the rancid smell will be immediately obvious. Some carrier oils like jojoba or olive oil will solidify in the fridge, so it is acceptable to keep them in a cool, dark area like a cupboard or a cabinet, instead.

CHAPTER 3

24 Pregnancy-safe Essential Oils

I HAVE TO say it; I am holding my hands up and admitting it - I have a love affair with essential oils! My life improves when I am exposed to the aromatic delights of one of nature's most beautiful gifts. My senses are enlivened, my endorphins soar, and the muscles of my face relax, sending forth a smile each and every time I open my precious little bottles of pure plant essence. Yes indeed, they are treasure to me!

It is with great joy then that I share with you, that which I hold very dear, in this chapter. Using essential oils in pregnancy can be wonderfully rewarding, and I will list and detail the beautiful essential oils that I use when working with my pregnant clients. It is an excellent list to refer to because the oils that are included can address many of the discomforts or conditions that might accompany your pregnancy and using these oils may improve your pregnancy wellness in some way. I also want to add that yes, there are other essential oils that are safe and effective to use in pregnancy, but even as an aromatherapist, I do not stray too far from this list when I am working with my pregnant clients.

When using essential oils, it is important to know their botanical name as well as the common, everyday name. This is because there are many different species of plants, and some go by the same common name but are in fact completely different plants with a different chemical make-up.

I would really like to emphasise the importance of proper dilution and dosage when using essential oils, and I encourage you to refer often to chapter 2 where you will find the quick blending guide. I know it may sometimes feel that you are using extremely small amounts of essential oils and that it cannot possibly be doing anything positive, or having any therapeutic effect, but be assured that it is.

DO NOT USE ESSENTIAL OILS NEAT/UNDILUTED. If being applied to the skin, or used in the bath, they must ALWAYS be diluted in a carrier oil - (unless otherwise stated in a very few cases).

So, here they are - 24 essential oils to help ease you through your pregnancy:

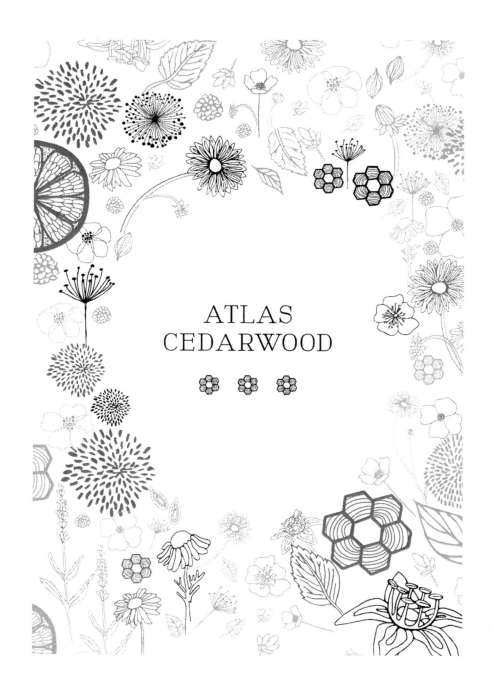

ATLAS
CEDARWOOD

1. ATLAS CEDARWOOD   Botanical Name: Cedrus atlantica

The cedarwood oil that we use in aromatherapy comes from the Cedrus atlantica tree which is known as a 'true cedar'. There are other 'false cedar' species like Red Cedarwood and Texas Cedarwood, which are from a different plant family, have a different chemical make-up, and actually come with contraindications if their essential oils were to be used. Cedrus atlantica, however, is grown in Morocco, and the oil is steam distilled from the wood chippings, or stumps of the trees. It has a gorgeously warm, sweet, and woody smell and it develops beautifully in a blend. It is known to help with conditions of the chest such as bronchitis, coughs, and asthma, and is also beneficial when treating stress if it manifests in the likes of shallow breathing or palpitations. This can be particularly useful in pregnancy if you are feeling stressed, or experiencing any sense of body/mind disconnect.

Atlas cedarwood is also really useful if you are lacking in confidence, which can sometimes be the case as your pregnancy progresses and your birthing comes closer. It also lends its sense of strength and expansiveness beautifully, while encouraging deep rootedness and grounding when you need it in your labour experience.

Properties of Atlas Cedarwood	Blending note	Blends well with
Encourages blood flow to the skin Expectorant Euphoric Grounding	Base	Frankincense Geranium Lemon Rose Sandalwood Sweet orange

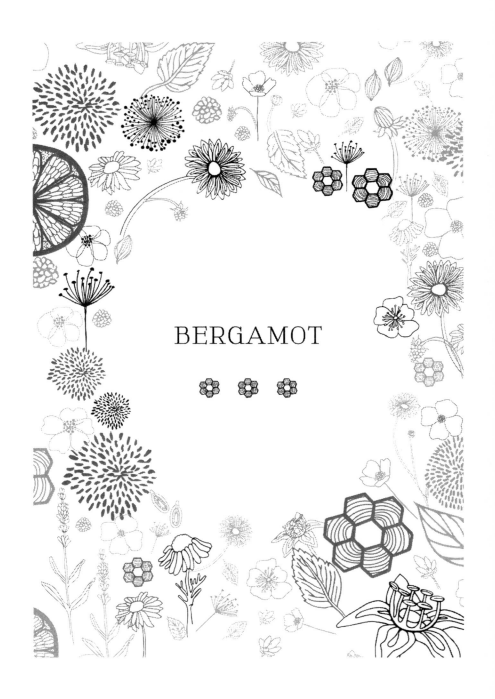

BERGAMOT

2. BERGAMOT   Botanical Name: Citrus aurantium/ Citrus bergamia

Bergamot is a beautifully fragrant citrus essential oil that is uplifting and refreshing. It takes its name from the town of Bergamo in Northern Italy, and traditionally, bergamot has been used in Italian folk medicine. It has also been used widely in the perfume industry for many years, and the bergamot tree is cultivated not for its fruit, which is thought too bitter for consumption, but for its beautiful essential oil. You are probably already familiar with bergamot as it is also used to fragrance Earl Grey tea, giving it its beautiful and distinctive aroma. Gorgeous!

In pregnancy, bergamot is useful because it is especially good for the treatment of urinary tract infections (UTIs), and is helpful in clearing up unusual vaginal discharge or cystitis. Due to its antiviral properties, bergamot can be used safely in the treatment of cold sores. Furthermore, it is a wonderful essential oil to use in skin care creams and lotions because of its benefits in healing the skin.

Properties of Bergamot	Blending note	Blends well with
Antidepressant	Top	Cardamom
Antifungal		Geranium
Antiseptic		Grapefruit
Antiviral		Lavender
Deodorising		Lemon
Fever-reducing		Rose
Pain-relieving		Sandalwood
Wound-healing		Sweet orange
		Ylang ylang

CAUTIONS: Bergamot, while very beneficial in skin care, ironically, can also increase the skin's likelihood of burning when exposed to UV rays, when used in dilutions of greater than 10 drops per 100ml of leave-on products. Please do not expose your skin to sunlight or UV rays for 12 hours should you be using bergamot in quantities greater than this. Therefore, use fewer than 10 drops of bergamot/100ml product, or use it in night time preparations.

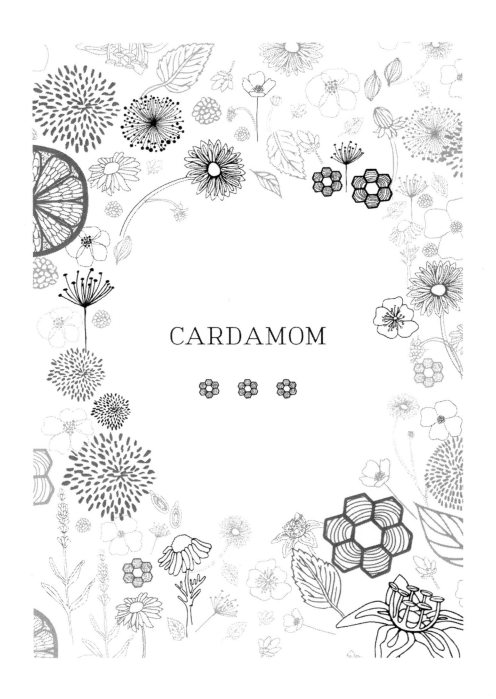

CARDAMOM

3. CARDAMOM Botanical Name: *Elettaria cardamomum*

Cardamom essential oil is a sweet and warm, spicy-toned essential oil that is distilled from the ripe fruits of the leafy cardamom shrub. Most commonly known as a condiment in Indian food, and as an aide in Eastern traditional medicine, history records it as also being used in incenses and perfumes. It has a distinctive, warm, rich aroma.

In pregnancy, I like to use cardamom for its carminative properties because it can help with queasiness and indigestion. It is known to settle the stomach and can be helpful in easing the sensation of nausea.

Properties of Cardamom	Blending note	Blends well with
Antiseptic Antispasmodic Expectorant Improves digestion Reduces flatulence Reduces fluid Stimulant	Middle	Bergamot Frankincense Lemon Sweet orange

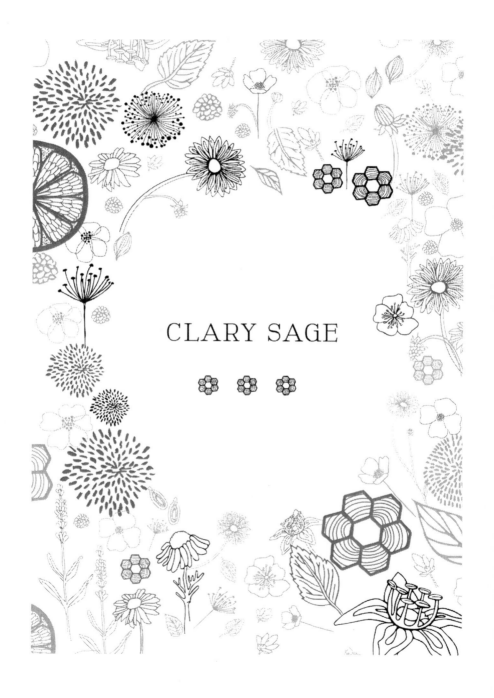

CLARY SAGE

4. CLARY SAGE   Botanical Name: *Salvia sclarea*

For me, clary sage is a bit like Marmite - you either love it or you hate it. It has a sweet yet sharp smell, with a dusty muskiness to it, which some people liken to hay. Many find its fragrance appealing, whereas others say that they find it somewhat overpowering.

In my experience, clary sage is a very powerful essential oil, it is often referred to as having euphoric properties and anecdotally, people have reported having hallucinogenic experiences when using it. Furthermore, while some texts may say that it is oestrogenic and can cause oestrogen-like reactions, in actuality there is no evidence to suggest a structural similarity between the molecules of clary sage constituents and those of oestrogen found in the human body.[5] Therefore, it is very unlikely to act like oestrogen in the body.

That being said, I still prefer to leave it to be used in labour, and not during the previous weeks of pregnancy.

(Outside of pregnancy, despite its lack of oestrogenic evidence, it may help to regulate scanty periods, or ease painful periods, and interestingly, it may play a helpful role in addressing post-natal depression.)

Clary sage can be useful in labour as it is strongly relaxing, and anti-spasmodic, thereby helping to reduce the discomfort of painful or unproductive contractions in labour. I find it is best to blend it with other essential oils, both in terms of improving its overall scent appeal, and also to temper its strength somewhat.

---

[5] P254 Essential Oil Safety, 2nd Ed. Tisserand and Young

Properties of Clary Sage	Blending note	Blends well with
Antispasmodic Aphrodisiac Euphoric Hormone regulator Lowers blood pressure Sedative	Top	Bergamot Lavender Lemon Rosewood Sandalwood

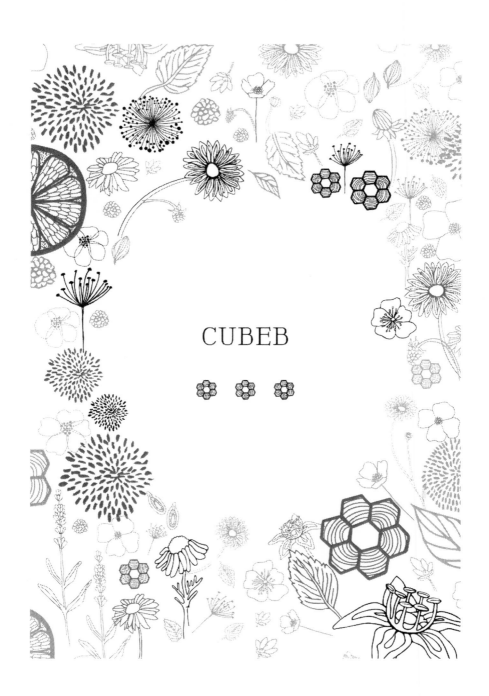

CUBEB

5. CUBEB   Botanical Name: *Piper cubeba*

Warm and spicy, but of a milder fragrance than the likes of black pepper, cubeb has been used in ayurvedic medicine and also to fight infection before the widespread use of antibiotics. It works well to ease conditions of the urinary and genital tract and therefore would be useful if you are suffering from UTIs in pregnancy. It is also helpful in addressing respiratory conditions such as chronic bronchitis, and also great at relieving muscular aches and pains, so it is a wonderful addition to the bath when blended with lavender and frankincense. It is also useful for indigestion and it may help to ease constipation and encourage proper bowel movement if blended and applied to the abdomen, or used as part of a blend for a bath.

Properties of Cubeb	Blending note	Blends well with
Antiviral Reduces flatulence Immune stimulant (especially for respiratory and urogenital conditions)	Middle	Bergamot Frankincense Grapefruit Lavender Neroli Sweet orange

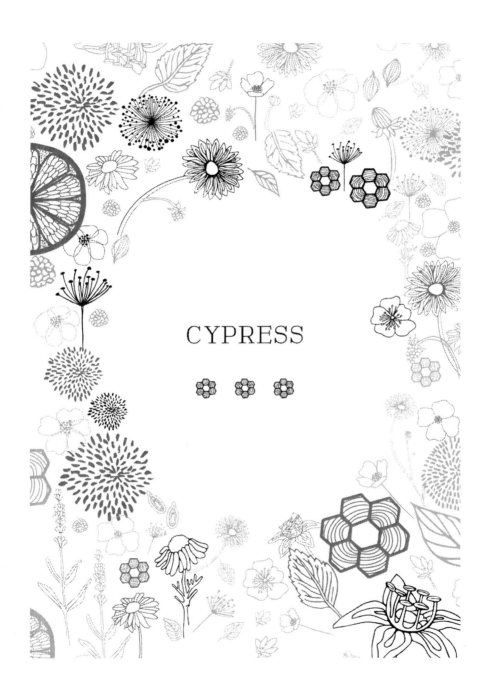

CYPRESS

6. CYPRESS   Botanical Name: *Cupressus sempervivens*

A fresh yet earthy and dry smelling oil that is distilled from the leaves, twigs, and cones of a tall evergreen tree. It is restorative and calming and is known to dry up areas, or situations, where there is excessive fluid involved.

Cypress is one of my go-to oils for both swelling of the legs and feet, and also varicose veins and haemorrhoids. It is also very good for excessive perspiration which may occur both during pregnancy and also after your baby has been born, as your body gets rid of the extra fluid it has gathered in pregnancy. It can help to contract the walls of blood vessels which is beneficial for anyone suffering from circulatory problems as this helps blood vessels to work more efficiently, providing better blood flow around the body.

Properties of Cypress	Blending note	Blends well with
Antiseptic Astringent Deodorising Reduces fluid Helpful in raising low blood pressure	Middle	Bergamot Geranium Grapefruit Lavender Lemon Rose

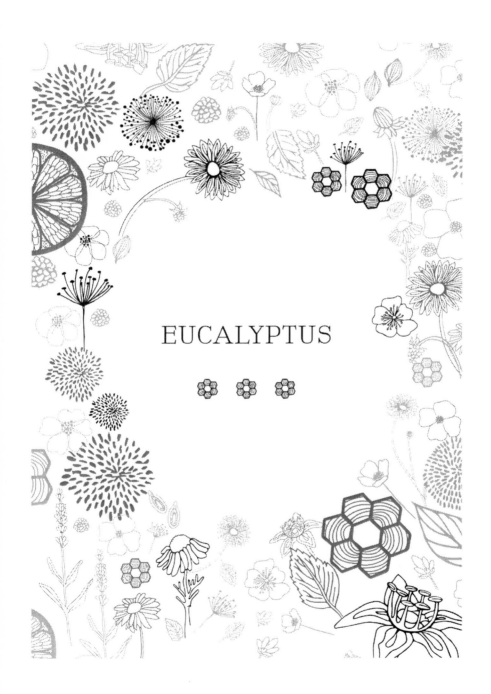

EUCALYPTUS

7. EUCALYPTUS   Botanical Name: *Eucalyptus globulus*

(There are different types of eucalyptus, but the most commonly available one is Eucalyptus globulus.)

Eucalyptus can be described as having a medicinal smell, with strong, fresh 'green' notes. It is strongly antiseptic and comes from distilling the leaves of the eucalyptus tree, which is native to Australia, although other countries such as China and Portugal now grow eucalyptus trees for their oil. It blends well with citrus and floral essential oils and is a wonderful oil in helping with infection and for upper respiratory conditions like the common cold, sinusitis, and bronchitis.

In pregnancy, using eucalyptus essential oil can help to improve upper respiratory conditions like bronchitis, asthma, coughs, colds, sinusitis, and throat infections. It is an overall immune stimulant, so can be very useful to vaporise around your home if you feel you're coming down with something. Eucalyptus oil is a safe alternative to use instead of normal over-the-counter cold and flu remedies that may not be recommended in pregnancy. However, one of its main constituents, (called 1,8-cineole), can cause breathing difficulties and problems of the central nervous system in young children, so it should not be applied to, or near the face of infants or children under the age of ten[6].

Eucalyptus is also known as a topical circulation stimulant (TCS), in that it improves blood flow to an area when applied topically to the skin, and therefore is beneficial in easing muscular aches and pains.

Properties of Eucalyptus	Blending note	Blends well with
Antiseptic Expectorant Immune stimulant	Top	Frankincense Grapefruit Lavender Lemon

---

[6] P273 Essential Oil Safety, 2nd Edition, Tisserand and Young, 2014

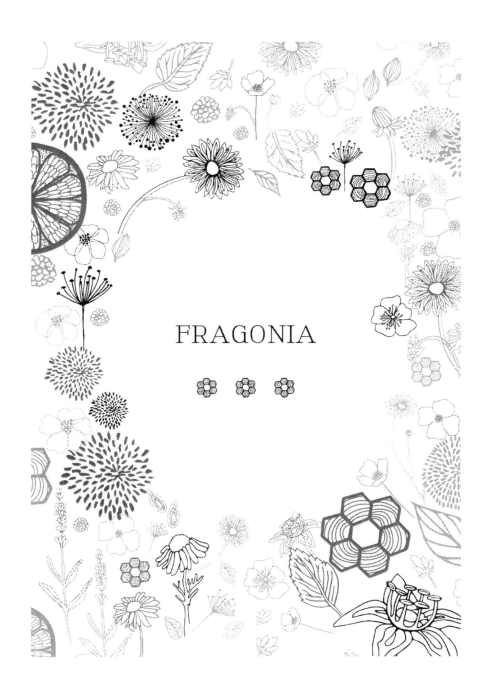

FRAGONIA

8. FRAGONIA   Botanical name: *Agonis fragrans*

The *Agonis fragrans* plant is a woody shrub that is native to Western Australia, and the essential oil is derived through the steam distillation of its twigs and leaves. Fragonia essential oil is similar to tea tree's antimicrobial action, but its fragrance is less medicinal, more lemony sherbet, and gentler in nature. It is truly a delightful essential oil to use, and its reported benefits include being a highly effective anti-depressant, a hormone regulator and an immune tonic with a special affinity for the respiratory system. It also has pain-relieving properties, helping to alleviate muscular aches and pains. Furthermore, there are reports of how well it can assist in the letting go of old, negative emotional blockages, and how it can promote relaxation, stress relief, and encourage a sense of happiness.

Properties of Fragonia	Blending note	Blends well with
Expectorant	Middle	Cubeb
Hormone regulator		Geranium
Immune stimulant		Grapefruit
Emotional balancer		Lavender
Pain relieving		Patchouli
Uplifting and cheerful		Roman chamomile
		Rose

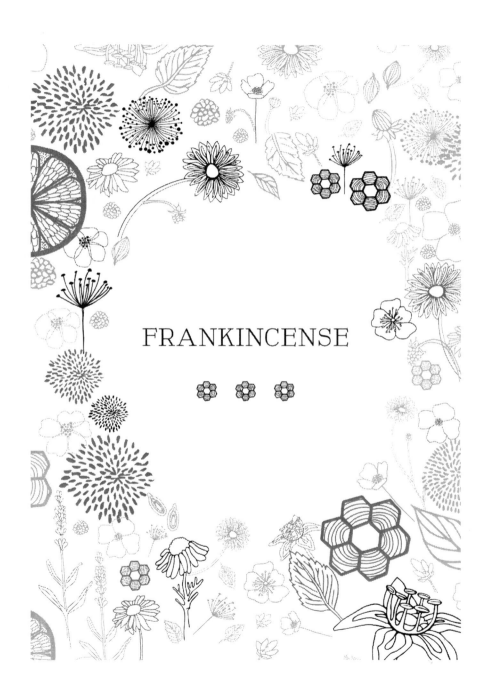

FRANKINCENSE

9. FRANKINCENSE   Botanical Name: *Boswellia carterii*

Fabulous frankincense! This is such a gorgeous essential oil, and has strong historical ties to sacred ceremonies and rituals. It was even one of the gifts brought by the three wise men for the birth of Jesus Christ. The essential oil is harvested from the *Boswellia carterii* tree which is mostly grown in northern Africa, and when little cuts are made in the bark, it releases beautiful, tear-like, resin drops, which are then steam-distilled to produce the essential oil. It is interesting to note that the resin tears appear in response to the bark being perforated, because frankincense is known to be helpful in wound-healing, in that it is rejuvenating and helps in the healing of broken or scarred skin. Consequently, frankincense is beautiful to use in skincare preparations because of its healing and restorative nature. It is also wonderful for addressing respiratory, or chest and lung imbalances as it can encourage deep breathing and a sense of meditative calm.

In pregnancy, frankincense would be very useful in helping you to keep calm should anxiety arise, or if you suffer from panic attacks. It improves circulation and therefore is also wonderful at easing aching, tired and tense muscles; it is ideal in a massage or a bath blend. Frankincense is also one of my favourite essential oils to use in a labour blend, given its calming and supportive nature. Later in the book, I gave details on specific oils and blends for labour, and frankincense features among them.

Properties of Frankincense	Blending note	Blends well with
Calming Meditative Encourages deep breathing Wound-healing Encourages blood flow to the skin	Middle	Atlas cedarwood Geranium Grapefruit Lavender Mandarin Roman chamomile Rose Rosewood Sweet orange

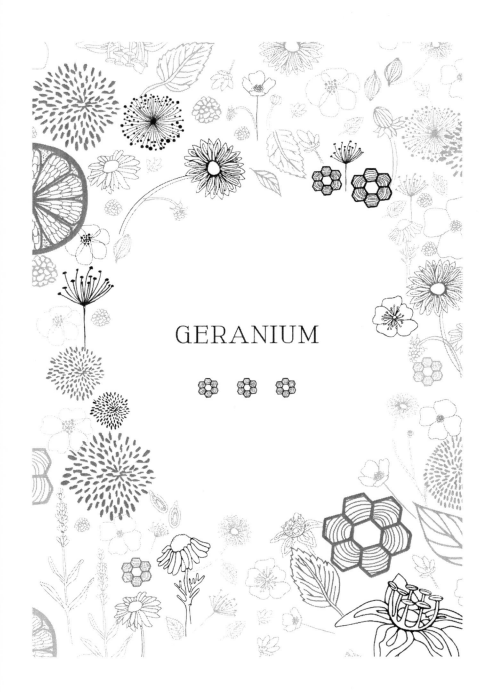

GERANIUM

10. GERANIUM   Botanical Name: *Pelargoinium graveolans*

Despite its name, the geranium used in aromatherapy is not the typical little red-flowered house plant that you see in your granny's porch. And here we realise the importance of knowing a plant's botanical name because the red-flowering houseplant is called *Pelargonium*, and while of the same family, the most common geranium used in aromatherapy is called *Pelargonium graveolans*. (This is also sometimes referred to as rose geranium, despite the fact that it is unrelated to rose essential oil.) Geranium essential oil is obtained by the steam distillation of the aromatic green parts of the plant, mostly the leaves, and perhaps surprisingly, the flowers are not used for the essential oil production. Some of the best geranium essential oil is produced in Egypt, but it is also grown in most other North African countries.

I really love using geranium essential oil; it has a beautiful floral fragrance and has many wonderful properties which make it very versatile. It is very useful when working with skin issues, as it can help to heal wounds and encourage new skin growth. It also has antiseptic and antiviral properties which are helpful when the oil is applied onto the tingling threat of a cold sore. Geranium is very balancing, and works its wonders on the skin because it can help to clear up areas of acne or imbalance.

It is brightening in nature because it improves a gloomy mood and also helps to balance hormones. It has diuretic properties, and in pregnancy that will help to reduce excess fluid in tired, tight, and swollen feet and ankles.

Properties of Geranium	Blending note	Blends well with
Antiviral Harmonising Hormone regulator Mood balancer Relaxing	Middle	Atlas cedarwood Frankincense Grapefruit Lavender Neroli Roman chamomile Sweet orange Ylang ylang

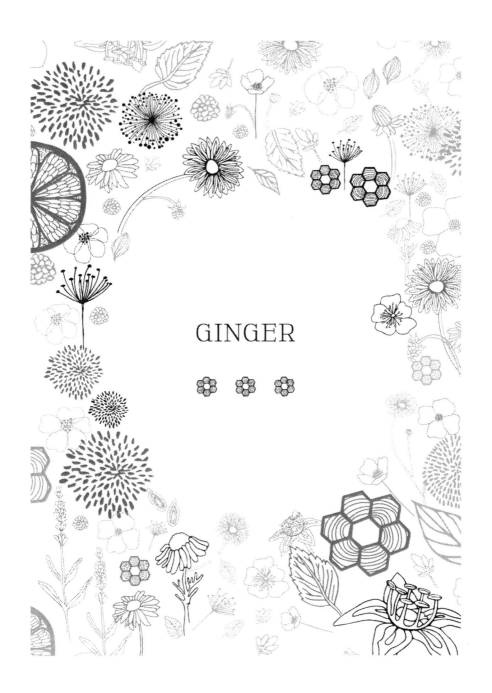

GINGER

11. GINGER   Botanical Name: *Zingiber officinale*

Ginger has been used in various cultures for many years and has become well known all over the world as a spice that is used for both culinary and health purposes. Its distinctive flavour makes for tasty curries, stir-fries, and tonics, and was thought to have originated in India. However, nowadays, it is probably best known in Chinese and Japanese cultures and plays a major role in traditional medicine in stimulating the immune system.

Ginger essential oil is distilled from the parts of the plant that grow underground, and not the tall reed-like branches that grow above ground, giving it an earthy and perhaps 'dusty' smell.

It is important never to use ginger essential oil neat on the skin, or undiluted in the bath as direct contact with the skin has been known to cause quite aggressive skin irritation. The essential oil can, of course, be diluted appropriately in any number of pure vegetable oils - preferably organic and cold-pressed.

In pregnancy, ginger may be used to address morning sickness and nausea, and to ease digestive stomach cramps. This can be in the form of ginger tea, or blending the essential oil to be used in a bath or massage oil blend. Unfortunately, not all pregnancy-related nausea will be alleviated this way. If you use ginger essential oil in your blends, and your nausea feels worse, then please discontinue its use.

Ginger is also excellent at improving the discomfort of aches and pains and can be used in a muscle rub blend to improve circulation and stiffness. This could also be used in the bath.

Properties of Ginger	Blending note	Blends well with
Reduces digestive cramps and spasms Encourages warming of the skin and increased blood flow at the skin's surface	Middle	Atlas cedarwood Lemon Mandarin Sandalwood Sweet orange

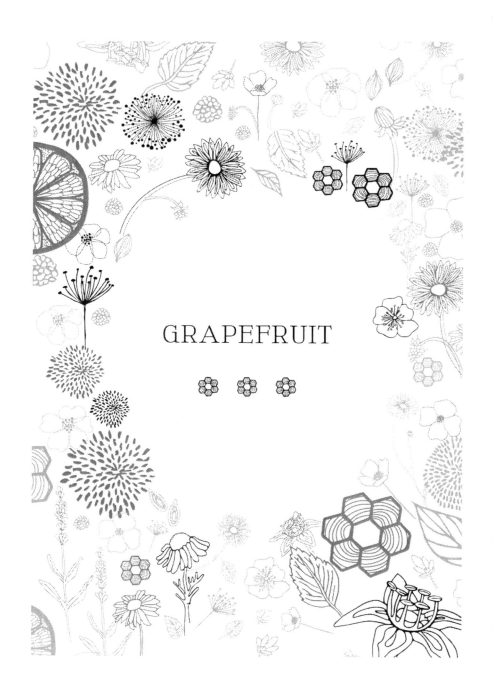

GRAPEFRUIT

12. GRAPEFRUIT   Botanical name: *citrus paradisi*

Like its botanical name infers, grapefruit does smell as if it hails from paradise. Its beautiful fragrance will invoke cheerfulness on even the darkest days, and spreads happiness and a feeling of brightness wherever it is used. It can help to improve a congested lymphatic system and in pregnancy, if you are suffering from swollen or puffy feet and ankles, grapefruit is excellent to include in a blend to massage into these problematic areas as it will help to shift the excess fluid that is gathering. Grapefruit is good at removing unwanted toxins from the body and is helpful as a liver tonic. When massaged in a blend into the abdominal and back area, it may improve sluggish digestion and help ease the discomfort of indigestion, and when applied to the face in skincare products, it has been known to improve the appearance of oily skin and breakouts. It is also useful in boosting the immune system and can be used in a vaporiser around the home, or even inhaled by putting one drop on a tissue, to help stop a head-cold from becoming fully blown. It is a wonderful daytime oil to use in body products or in the bath due to its refreshing and uplifting qualities.

Properties of Grapefruit	Blending note	Blends well with
Antispasmodic Cheering Removes excess fluid Immune stimulant Uplifting	Top	Most oils but especially Cypress Frankincense Geranium Rose Ylang ylang

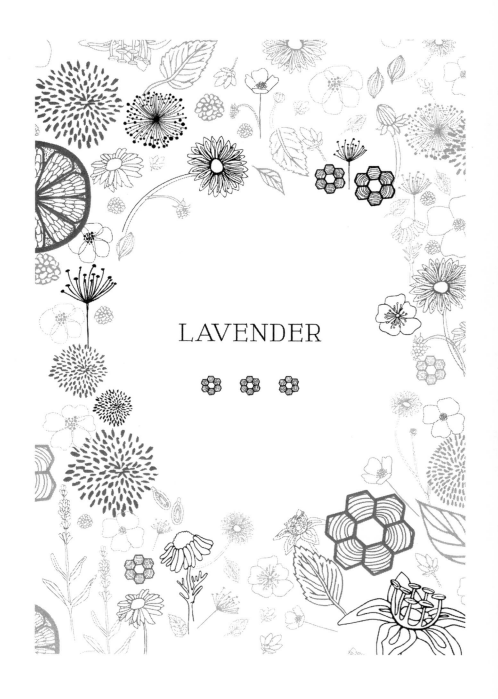

LAVENDER

13. LAVENDER   Botanical name: *Lavandula angustifolia*

Where do we start with lavender? I know that lavender essential oil is used in so many things, but to be quite honest, it's because it has such beautiful properties and can help in a great variety of ways. I think it's safe to say that it would feature on my desert island list of essential oils!

It has a beautiful floral fragrance and often evokes in people vivid memories of loved ones they knew or places they have been. Probably best known for its relaxing properties, lavender also has pain relieving properties which make it great at easing common pregnancy aches and pains. Calming and soothing, lavender can induce sleepiness, but it can also have the opposite effect to the desired one if you use too much, in that it can keep you awake. Another example would be if you were using lavender to help lift a headache, but if you use too much, it can actually make your headache worse. Hence, always remember the importance of proper usage and dilution when using essential oils.

Lavender can also be applied to insect bites, stings, and minor burns.

Properties of Lavender	Blending note	Blends well with
Pain relieving Antimicrobial Reduces cramps and spasms in the digestive system Calming Comforting Skin healing Floral Healing Lowers blood pressure Relaxing	Middle	Most oils but especially Atlas cedarwood Frankincense Geranium Neroli Roman chamomile Rose

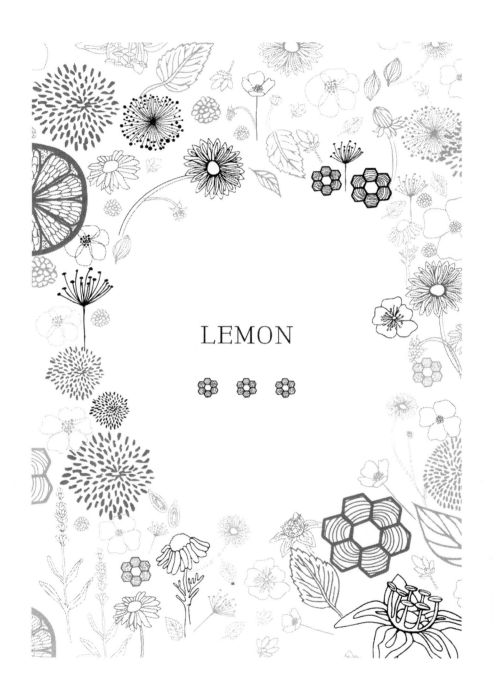

LEMON

14. LEMON   Botanical name: *Citrus limonum*

Another beautiful, bright smelling citrus essential oil, lemon is steam distilled from the rind of the lemon fruit. Everyone knows the zesty fragrance of lemon, and it seems to be universally appealing. As well as being delightfully fragrant, lemon essential oil is also wonderful at boosting the immune system, and like grapefruit, it is really good at helping to ward off colds and flu. It is also very effective in helping to reduce swelling and puffiness as it is a diuretic and promotes improved functioning of the lymphatic system, keeping both mum and baby happy. You can use lemon essential oil to great avail in skin care preparations if you have oily or congested skin, due to its astringent properties. Furthermore, lemon is excellent when used in a vaporiser around the home as a room freshener; it will do a much better job at shifting unwanted odours, and is healthier for you and your baby than the artificial fragrances found in mainstream air fresheners and scented candles which are actually hormone disrupters.

Properties of Lemon	Blending note	Blends well with
Antidepressant	Top	Cardamom
Antimicrobial		Geranium
Antiviral		Grapefruit
Bright		Lavender
Cheery		Mandarin
Immune stimulant		Neroli
Removes excess fluid		Patchouli
Uplifting		Rose
		Vetiver

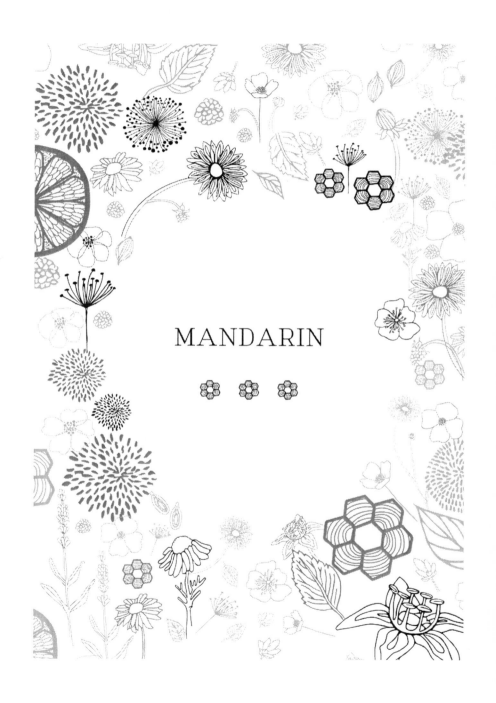

MANDARIN

15. MANDARIN Botanical name: *Citrus reticulata Blanco*

Mandarin essential oil is also classified as a citrus oil. However, like its fruit, it is much sweeter and milder in nature than the likes of grapefruit or lemon. It is also produced from the steam distillation of its rind. Mandarin essential oil has a very soothing quality and can work wonders when used in a vaporiser or oil burner to calm an anxious or upset state of mind. It is gorgeous in skin care preparations, and because of its skin-healing and regenerative benefits, can be helpful in addressing stretch marks or skin irritations.

Properties of Mandarin	Blending note	Blends well with
Antidepressant	Top	Frankincense
Calming		Geranium
Comforting		Lavender
Digestive tonic		Neroli
Gentle		Roman chamomile
Skin healing		Rose
Soothing		Sweet orange

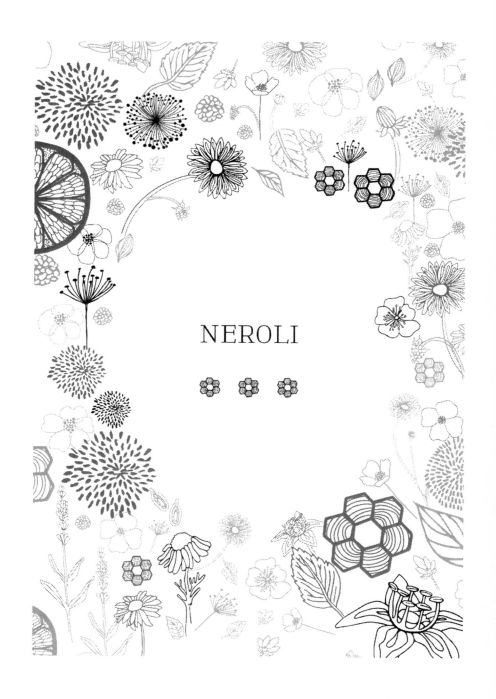

NEROLI

16. NEROLI   Botanical name: *Citrus aurantium var. Amara*

Neroli, or orange blossom, is often referred to as being a precious essential oil, as it requires the steam distillation of many tonnes of the orange flower heads to produce even a small amount of the oil. This is reflected in the very high price of neroli essential oil. However, despite its expense, it has been a favourite in the perfume industry for centuries because it has such a beautiful fragrance, and it certainly adds luxury to any blend. However, neroli oil is not just a pretty face, in that it has many therapeutic benefits as well (think of it as the over-achiever in the class!), such as the ability to calm and soothe, and to relieve stress. It is very useful if you suffer from pregnancy insomnia and it can also be used with great success in helping to lift a depressed mood, or to calm a panic attack.

I do not often use neroli in an oil burner or vaporiser due to its expense, however, I love to use it in an oil blend for massage, the bath, or in face creams and body lotions. When used in the evening time, it can help to overcome insomnia, and in addition, it promotes skin-healing and is wonderful in improving the look and feel of your skin. In pregnancy, it is excellent when used in body preparations to help reduce the appearance of stretch marks and scars, and also in the treatment of fine lines and facial wrinkles. You may also have seen orange flower water, which is the hydrosol of neroli, for sale as a facial tonic. This is beautiful to use on the skin due to its mild astringent properties, but is much lighter and can be used more liberally than the essential oil.

Post-natally, neroli may be useful in helping to balance the peaks and troughs of hormones and emotions, and to support you in your weeks and months of early motherhood.

Properties of Neroli	Blending note	Blends well with
Antidepressant Antispasmodic Calming Sedative Skin-healing	Middle	Geranium Lavender Mandarin Patchouli Rosewood Sandalwood Sweet orange

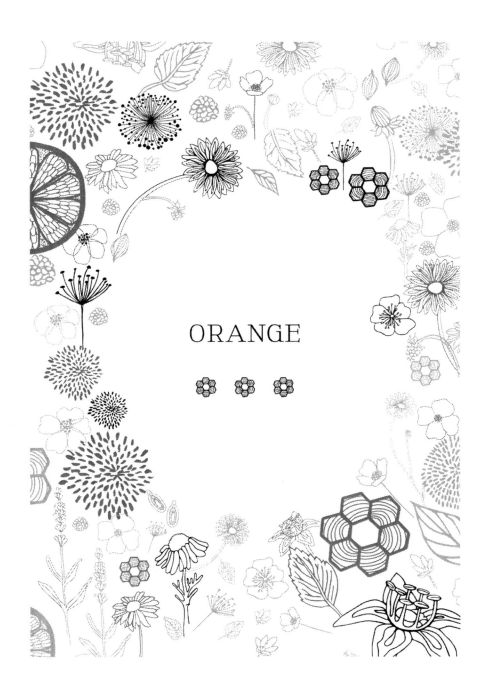

ORANGE

17. ORANGE (SWEET)   Botanical Name: *Citrus Sinensis*

Who doesn't love the smell of fresh oranges being peeled? That's the fragrance of sweet orange essential oil, and like its other citrus sisters, sweet orange is also steam distilled from the rinds of the orange fruit. I feel it is a good idea to choose citrus oils that come from an organically grown crop, given that the essential oil is harvested from the skin, and how we don't want to be distilling pesticides as well.

Sweet orange essential oil is superb at dispelling gloominess and lifting a depressed mood; it can also calm nervous tension and help to settle anxiety, which many women can suffer from in their pregnancy. They may worry about their pregnancy going ok, or if their developing baby will be healthy and well. Sweet orange can be very supportive at these times and can easily be vaporised around your home, or inhaled directly from a tissue (1 or 2 drops on a tissue is sufficient).

Sweet orange is also used beautifully in skin care, both for its appealing fragrance and its myriad benefits, which include its ability to help balance oiliness and to unclog congested pores.

Sweet orange essential oil is beneficial if you're experiencing excessive flatulence in pregnancy, and is also known as a digestive tonic. Furthermore, something which is of particular relevance in pregnancy, is that it is helpful in promoting proper bowel function and in easing digestive discomfort. Sweet orange, blended with cardamom and peppermint, and massaged into the abdomen and lower back may prove helpful in relieving the discomfort of constipation. This blend could also be applied to the feet and hands, and used with reflexology.

Properties of Sweet Orange	Blending note	Blends well with
Antidepressant Antispasmodic Astringent Digestive tonic Lowers blood pressure Uplifting (mood)	Top	Most oils but especially Cardamom Cubeb Ginger Mandarin Neroli Patchouli Peppermint Roman chamomile Rose

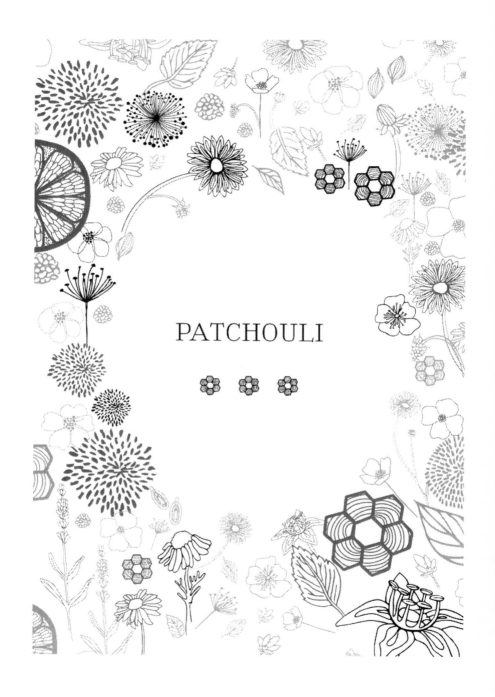

PATCHOULI

18. PATCHOULI Botanical name: *Pogostemon cablin*

Patchouli oil is steam distilled from the leaves and stems of the *Pogostemon cablin* shrub which is grown for its oil mainly in Indonesia and Malaysia, as well as China and India. Patchouli is lovely in blends, and only a little is needed to have an effect. It is very good at resolving body/mind disconnect, for calming nervous exhaustion, and for reducing stress. It is also good in addressing skin conditions like eczema, and sore, and inflamed skin. Due to its strong, earthy nature, I like to use it in situations where someone needs more grounding or finds themselves to be too much in their heads and in need of a renewed sense of connectedness.

It has quite a heavy fragrance, and I feel that it is overpowering if used by itself. However, it mixes fantastically and lends depth and substance to the overall fragrance of your blend. In pregnancy, I find it to be very helpful in letting go of stress and tension, perhaps in a blend for the bath, or a massage oil at the end of a long day to help encourage a better night's sleep.

Properties of Patchouli	Blending note	Blends well with
Antidepressant	Base	Geranium
Comforting		Grapefruit
Skin healing		Lavender
Diuretic		Mandarin
Earthy		Rose
Grounding		Sandalwood
Musky		Sweet orange
Peaty		

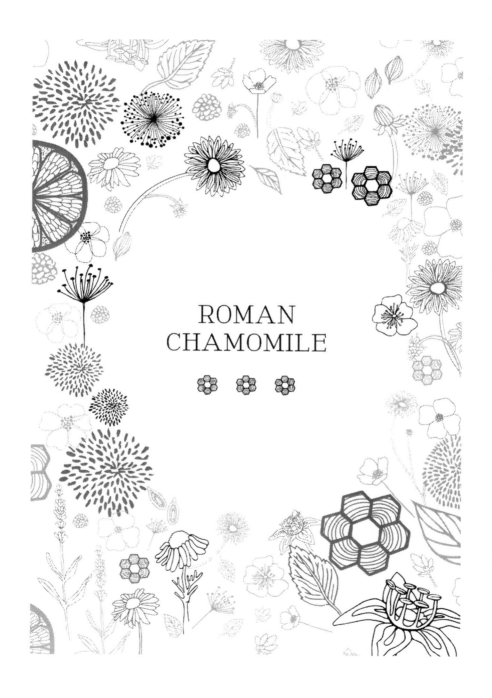

ROMAN
CHAMOMILE

19. ROMAN CHAMOMILE   Botanical name: *Anthemis nobilis*

The joy of roman chamomile! This essential oil is distilled from the lovely white flowering tops of the chamomile herb and is equally lovely in smell. In Spanish, its name is Manzanilla, which means 'little apple' and it certainly has a beautifully sweet, almost apple-like aroma. Roman chamomile might also feature in my desert island list of essential oils because it has so many beneficial properties and is versatile in blends. It is calming and restorative in nature both for body and mind, and you can only feel happier with having inhaled its beautiful fragrance. It is known to promote more restful sleep and is also helpful at easing aches and pains.

When used in skin creams or balms, it can help soothe broken or inflamed skin and is well known for its healing properties. Roman chamomile is also helpful in balancing the digestive system, and chamomile tea is wonderful when taken after a heavy meal.

Properties of Roman Chamomile	Blending note	Blends well with
Pain-relieving Anti-inflammatory Antispasmodic Calming Reduces flatulence Cheerful Comforting Digestive tonic Sedative	Middle	Frankincense Geranium Lavender Mandarin Neroli Rose Sweet orange Vetiver

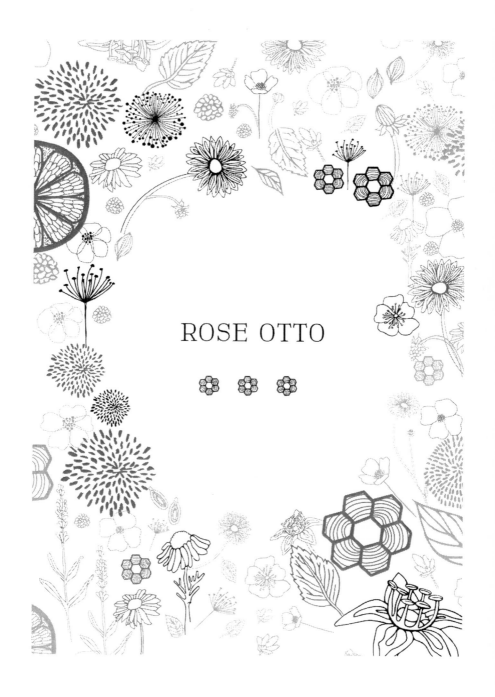

ROSE OTTO

20. ROSE OTTO   Botanical name: *Rosa damascena*

Warm, floral, and alluringly feminine, rose otto is a beautiful essential oil that is wonderful in supporting women throughout their various life stages. It is gorgeous in pregnancy skincare, and its anti-inflammatory and antibacterial nature will help to reduce redness and angry, inflamed skin – stretch marks included. Another wonderful benefit of using rose essential oil in your blends is that it can help to address any past emotional trauma and help to alleviate emotional heartache or stress. It may be useful in helping to heal from previous birth-related trauma where you have suffered post-traumatic stress syndrome.

The best rose oil comes from Bulgaria, and like neroli, it takes many tonnes of rose petals to make a few millilitres of rose essential oil. Unfortunately, because of this, it is one of the most, if not the most expensive essential oils to buy. The good news, however, is that you only need to use very little at any one time. Be aware of adulterated rose essential oil. If it is cheap to buy, it is not real rose otto oil and has probably had other components of less expensive essential oils added to it, like geranium. You will also come across pre-diluted rose essential oil which has been made to be about 6% dilution in the likes of jojoba carrier oil. This is ok to use for your own blends if you buy it from a reputable supplier, and certainly makes it more affordable. (Remember, it still needs to be further diluted in your own blends for safe use in pregnancy.)

Properties of Rose Otto	Blending note	Blends well with
Antibacterial	Base	Atlas cedarwood
Anti-inflammatory		Cubeb
Euphoric		Geranium
Heart tonic		Frankincense
Nurturing		Mandarin
		Lavender
		Lemon
		Neroli
		Sweet orange

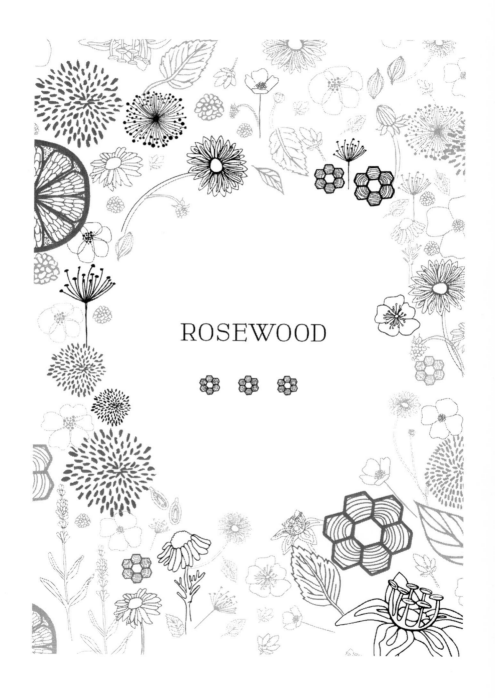

ROSEWOOD

21. ROSEWOOD   Botanical name: *Aniba rosaeodora*

Rosewood is another very special oil, and one that has of late been at the centre of ethical and environmental debate. Given that the beautiful rosewood trees, which are native to tropical areas like Brazil, India and Madagascar, must be felled in order to obtain the oil from the wood chippings, there is obvious concern about environmental damage and the need for sustainable farming. Ethical companies are carrying out this sustainable rosewood farming by replacing older felled trees with younger saplings. Unfortunately, many areas have suffered extensive, illegal felling of rosewood forests, leaving some true rosewood species close to extinction. Bearing this in mind, I do not like to waste rosewood and only buy it from a credible, sustainable source.

Rosewood essential oil is prized because of its beautiful fragrance; it has been used in perfumery for centuries, and also for its health benefits because of its many therapeutic properties. It is marvellous at helping to reduce stress, and to boost the immune system especially in a period of recuperation or convalescence. It is fabulous in skincare preparations and, being non-irritant, while at the same time being antibacterial and antiseptic, it is good in addressing skin breakouts or acne.

Rosewood is also excellent at calming the mind and steadying nerves, and for this reason, I feel that it is wonderful to use in the later stages of pregnancy, and also in labour.

Properties of Rosewood	Blending note	Blends well with
Hypotensive	Middle	Atlas cedarwood
Immune tonic		Lavender
Sedative		Lemon
Skin healing		Mandarin
Supportive, especially in convalescence		Neroli
		Rose
Uplifting (mood)		Sandalwood
		Sweet orange

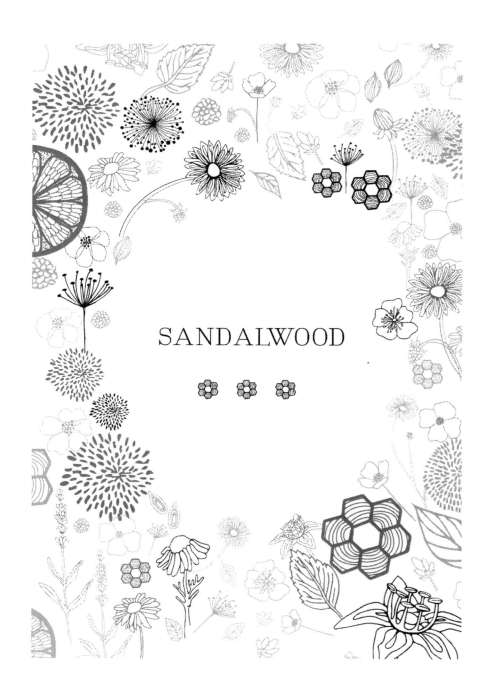

SANDALWOOD

22. SANDALWOOD Botanical name: *Santalum album*

Sandalwood oil, like rosewood, is obtained from the hardwood centre of the tree and therefore requires that the tree be felled to harvest it. There is a greater yield of essential oil from trees that are at least 30 years old, with even greater quantities being obtained from trees that have reached 50 or 60 years old. Therefore, the same ethical and environmental issues are at play regarding the sustainability of the harvesting methods and unfortunately, many of the *santalum album* trees are on the verge of extinction in their native India. However, New Zealand has emerged as a forerunner in the sustainable production of sandalwood oil as it is committed to the replanting of younger sandalwood trees to replace the older trees that have been used for their hardwood and essential oil. It is of course no surprise to learn that sandalwood essential oil has many physical and emotional benefits, and this is why it is so much in demand.

I feel that sandalwood is so special that it almost has a sacred feel to it, and its fragrance is gorgeously alluring with the oil having excellent grounding properties. In pregnancy, given that sandalwood is an adrenal tonic, it can be used to calm the body and the mind and is great to use if suffering from prolonged stress, e.g. work situations or strained family life. It is beautiful for skincare products given its rejuvenating properties, and is also good at addressing acne. It is also particularly useful in encouraging better body/mind connectedness

Thanks to its antimicrobial nature, sandalwood is helpful in treating throat or respiratory tract infections. It is useful in alleviating a sore throat if applied to the external area of the neck and throat and massaged in (Use 10ml of your preferred carrier oil and add three drops of sandalwood – apply two or three drops of the blend). Also, sandalwood can be helpful in addressing urinary tract infections, to which many women can succumb in pregnancy. This can be resolved by using sandalwood in a blend in the bath or as a massage oil, and applied to the lower abdomen, lower back, hip area, and tops of your legs.

Properties of Sandalwood	Blending note	Blends well with
Antimicrobial Grounding Relaxing Sedative Skin-healing Tonic - Urogenital/Adrenal	Base	Atlas cedarwood Cubeb Frankincense Lavender Mandarin Rose Sweet orange Vetiver

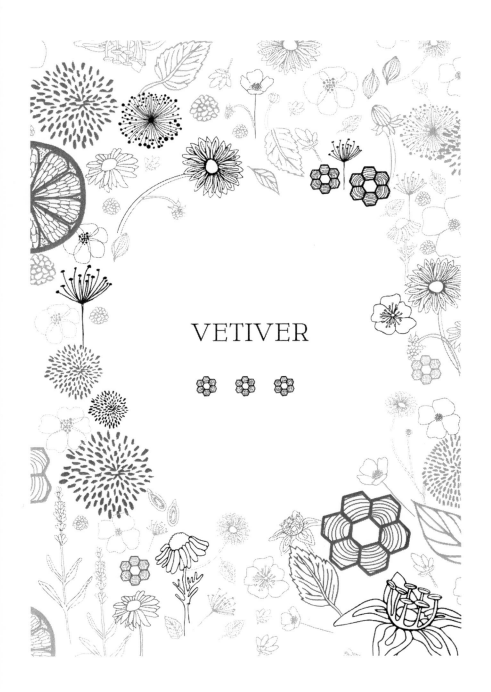

VETIVER

23. VETIVER   Botanical name: *Vetiveria zizanoides*

Using a blend with vetiver before bed can really improve your night's sleep and when used in the bath it will ease aches and pains, and tired legs, setting you up for sleepy heaven. It is very grounding for the body, but because it is so relaxing for the mind, it can leave you with a slightly spaced feeling, so it's definitely an evening time oil, and not one to use if you need to pay full attention to what you're doing, like driving. Vetiver is also especially good at helping to alleviate lower back pain.

If you're using it in the bath, you will also notice a positive effect on your skin if it is dry, or if you suffer from the likes of psoriasis, eczema or acne.

Given that it can help to slow rapid breathing and ease panic attacks, vetiver in pregnancy is particularly useful if you are prone to anxiety, or have any sense of fear, perhaps about your birthing experience or the health of your developing baby.

Properties of Vetiver	Blending note	Blends well with
Calming	Base	Bergamot
Grounding		Geranium
Pain-relieving (especially for lower back pain)		Frankincense
		Lavender
Relaxing		Lemon
Sedative		Rose
Slows rapid breathing		Sweet orange

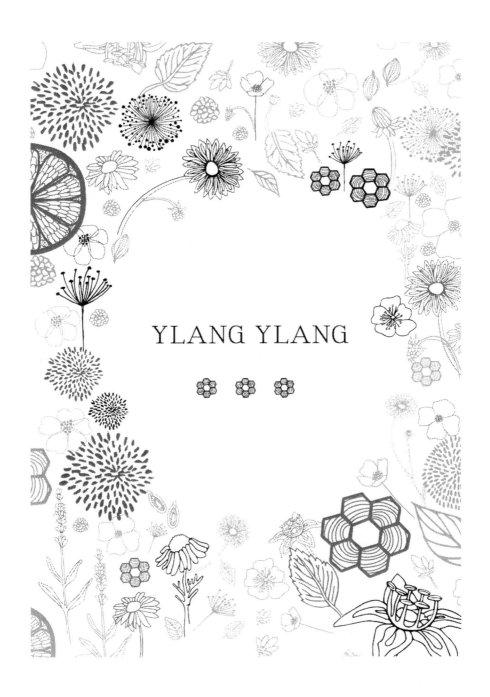

YLANG YLANG

24. YLANG YLANG   Botanical name: *Cananga odorata*

Ylang ylang is an exotic-smelling floral essential oil that can have a strong, distinctive fragrance by itself and is often referred to as being 'heady' in nature. However, blended with other lighter, top note essential oils, it is perfect in pregnancy in helping to lower high blood pressure*, address panic attacks, calm anxiety, and release tension.

The *cananga odorata* tree is native to the Philippines, but nowadays the oil is mostly sourced in Madagascar and the nearby island of Reunion, as well as Caribbean islands like Trinidad and the beautiful flowers are steam distilled to produce the essential oil.

*Please always consult your caregiver in pregnancy if you are suffering from elevated blood pressure, especially if it is sudden, and/or is accompanied by swelling in the feet, hands, face, and a headache.

Properties of Ylang ylang	Blending note	Blends well with
Alleviates anxiety Aphrodisiac Floral Lowers blood pressure Sedative Sweet	Base	Ginger Grapefruit Lavender Neroli Rosewood Sandalwood Sweet orange Make sure the amount of ylang ylang used **does not exceed 20 drops in 100ml.**

CHAPTER 4

Carrier Oils

PLANT OILS AND butters have been used for centuries all over the world for culinary, medicinal, and cosmetic purposes. They are nothing like mineral oil which is a by-product in the processing of crude oil to produce bitumen, gasoline, kerosene, and diesel, amongst other petroleum products.

They have played a central role in religious and sacred ceremonies and sometimes have been used as payment in exchange for goods or services. Forming a staple in day to day life, plant oils and butters have been used by ancient tribes, and great civilisations all over the world, and they have transcended the centuries and the continents to play an important role in our lives today. We use oils in and on our food, for taste and health benefits, and beauty benefits too. By applying them to the skin, we reap the benefits of their fatty content both on the outer layer of the skin and also, as they penetrate the skin's barrier and assimilate with the fatty lower layers of the skin.

Plant oils and butters are a valuable addition to our daily pregnancy routine, and here I will talk about how we can use them on your skin, drawing upon their health-enhancing characteristics in their own right. When buying your liquid oils, it is better to opt for ones that are labelled cold pressed and organic, and that come in dark bottles, preferably made of glass.

In the paragraphs that follow, I profile six different plant oils, and I have also included recipes for each oil, and how you can use it to help you in your pregnancy. However, you will also find more oil blends for pregnancy-related conditions in Chapter 6. Please note, the recipes for body oils can be used all over your body, but take care to avoid your eyes and mucous membranes.

None of the recipes is suitable for use on infants under three years due to the essential oil content.

1. CALENDULA Botanical name: *Calendula Officinalis*

Calendula oil comes from macerating the calendula flower heads in another vegetable oil, normally sunflower oil, to make calendula infusion. Often, there is an antioxidant like rosemary extract or vitamin E added to help lengthen the shelf life of the oil. I love using calendula oil in body products because it is a herb that has such well known skin-healing properties with its being anti-inflammatory, and soothing in nature.

Stretch-mark body oil with Calendula (100ml)

Calendula infusion 40ml
Sweet Almond oil 30ml
Rosehip oil 27ml
Vit. E 2ml

Add the following essential oils:
Bergamot 5 drops
Frankincense 6 drops
Geranium 4 drops
Lavender 8 drops
Patchouli 1 drop
Rose 1 drop

Apply a moderate amount of your blend once or twice daily to areas that may be prone to stretchmarks, or where stretchmarks may have already appeared. Massage in well.

2. COCONUT OIL Botanical name: *Cocos nuciferous*

Coconut oil comes from coconuts that grow on palm trees, generally in Asia or the West Indies. Given that these areas are susceptible to grand-scale deforestation and major destruction of natural habitat to make room for the likes of palm tree cultivation, it is a good idea to check how your coconut oil was sourced. When buying your coconut oil, choose one that is virgin and organic, and if possible one that is sustainably sourced. The planting of palm tree plantations in Southeast Asia often means that the natural habitat is being destroyed and native animals (you may have seen the distressing images of displaced or injured orangutans due to forests and natural ecosystems having been destroyed by fire) are losing their natural habitat and ecosystem.

Coconut oil generally comes in two forms:

Solid coconut oil (also known as coconut butter) which is normally packaged in a large tub, and fractionated coconut oil, which is a thin, clear liquid because it has had many of the solid fatty acids or long-chain triglycerides removed in processing, and will be packaged in bottles.

Solid coconut oil has all the distinctive, familiar fragrance of coconut and can be used in cooking as well as in beauty or health preparations. Fractionated coconut oil is a very light liquid in texture, is odourless and is good for combining with other cold-pressed vegetable oils for massage purposes. It also has a long shelf-life because it can stay good for 4-5 years (It's still best to store it in dark glass bottles away from direct light and heat sources).

Coconut oil is a really effective emollient for skin and hair care purposes and will leave your skin feeling very soft and supple. It has many benefits and positive actions on the body, and its popularity seems to be ever-increasing. I feel that it is better to use coconut in its unprocessed form as it contains all of the botanical components in their synergistic entirety. However, if you choose to use fractionated coconut oil in your preparations like the one I've suggested below, it is beneficial to blend it with other cold-pressed liquid vegetable oils before using it on your skin, to give it more comprehensive nourishment.

Conditioning Hair Oil with (Liquid Fractionated) Coconut Oil (100ml)

Coconut Oil 40ml
Sweet Almond Oil 35ml
Calendula Oil 23ml
Vitamin E 1ml

Add the following essential oils:
Atlas cedarwood 2 drops
Lavender 8 drops
Lemon 9 drops
Sweet orange 6 drops

After washing your hair massage a maximum of 15ml (depending on the length of your hair) of the oil blend through your hair and leave on for 30-45 minutes. Wash it out with a mild shampoo or, if you prefer, cover it with a shower cap (attractive, I know!) and leave on overnight, and then wash out in the morning.

3. SWEET ALMOND OIL Botanical name: *Prunus amygdalus dulcis*

Sweet Almond oil is a very versatile oil, and it is clear to light yellow in colour. It spreads easily and many massage therapists use it as a staple in their professional practice. It is mostly made up of oleic acid which is also known as Omega-9. Therefore, sweet almond oil is a good oil to use on your skin because oleic acid has anti-inflammatory properties which can help in keeping the skin in good condition and can improve skin healing. Oleic acid is also known to be regenerative and moisturising, and is also readily absorbed by the skin, which means that sweet almond oil is great in many facial and body preparations.

Dry Skin Body Oil with Sweet Almond (100ml)

Sweet Almond Oil 50ml
Thistle Oil 20ml
Sunflower Oil 15ml
Jojoba Oil 10ml
Vitamin E 2ml

Add the following essential oils:
Bergamot 6 drops
Frankincense 7 drops
Neroli 3 drops
Sweet orange 9 drops

This body oil can be used all over, but take care to avoid your eyes and mucous membranes. It is not suitable for infants under three years.

4.   GRAPESEED OIL   Botanical name: *Vitis vinifera*

Grapeseed is another very adaptable and versatile carrier oil, and is a perfect solution for anyone who suffers from nut allergies and wants to avoid any potential sources of allergens in nut-derived oils. While grapeseed feels like a light oil, it has many benefits for the body too. It is easily absorbed by the skin and therefore doesn't leave an overly sticky or 'oily' feel on your skin. It has a high linoleic acid, or Omega 6, content. This can be absorbed through the skin so that the whole body as well as the skin, benefits from the Omega 6. Grapeseed oil can be beneficial in supporting proper circulation, and this I feel, can be helpful if you suffer from the likes of swollen feet and ankles because by massaging these areas, the blood flow is improved and therefore the lymphatic system is also stimulated to help keep fluid moving.

If you would like a richer, more nourishing effect on your skin, grapeseed can be blended with the likes of sweet almond, or avocado oil, as these oils have a greater fatty content and lend extra nourishment to the skin. Grapeseed is a lovely oil to use on your face as it is helpful in addressing skin that is prone to oiliness or acne breakouts. It may also prove beneficial in reducing the appearance of enlarged pores.

Cold pressed, and organic grapeseed oil maintains the integrity of all the oil's essential nutrients, and is therefore, more beneficial in its use than the refined or heat processed version.

Toning Leg Oil with Grapeseed oil (100ml)

Grapeseed oil 80ml
Sweet Almond oil 10ml
Fractionated coconut oil 9ml

Add the following essential oils:
Cubeb 3 drops
Frankincense 6 drops
Grapefruit 8 drops
Lemon 6 drops
Sandalwood 2 drops

Apply a moderate amount of the blend to your legs in an upward motion and massage in well. Avoid any direct contact with varicose veins.

5. JOJOBA OIL Botanical name: *Simmondisia chinensis*

Jojoba oil comes from pressing the seeds of an evergreen bush that tends to grow in the Mexican, Arizona, and California desert and arid areas, and is actually more correctly categorised as a liquid wax, as opposed to a vegetable oil, (however, we will still continue to call it an oil). This makes it perfect in protecting the skin and increasing suppleness. Jojoba is often referred to as being similar in its makeup to that of our skin's sebum, and because of this, is excellent at re-balancing our skin's own oil production. It may sound a little counterintuitive to be putting oil on your skin in the hope of balancing it if you already have oily skin. However, your skin may be producing too much oil because it has been stripped of its natural lubrication by cosmetic products or preparations that were too harsh for your skin, or used ingredients that caused an imbalance in your skin's function. Consequently, it may be overcompensating by producing too much oil and making your skin feel greasy.

When you use a plant oil like jojoba, or a product made up of plant oils, and not mineral oil, your skin is given the chance to rebalance itself and reduce the excess production of sebum. The jojoba can mix perfectly with the skin's own sebum, and will not block the pores. This rebalancing process may take a few weeks, and it may feel worse before it feels better, but rest assured that your skin will look, feel, and function so much better if it is allowed to breathe properly, and is supported by good, nourishing ingredients.

Jojoba oil feels beautiful on the skin and is wonderful in addressing areas of inflammation (again, think stretch marks), dryness, and exposed areas. Due to its balancing nature, jojoba is excellent in the treatment of acne-prone skin. It also has anti-bacterial properties which can help to control the spread of bacteria that can cause breakouts and infection. There is no need to store your jojoba oil in the fridge as it is a very stable oil and does not easily degrade or go rancid. If however, you do store your oil in a cooler place, you will notice that it may solidify into a white mass. This is easily reversed by placing your bottle of now-solid oil into a bowl of warm water and waiting for it to melt. This does not affect the integrity of your oil, which can in fact stay good for about 4 to 5 years.

Acne-Prone Face Oil with Jojoba (100ml)

Jojoba Oil 20ml
Rosehip Seed Oil 20ml
Grapeseed Oil 40ml
Apricot Kernel Oil 19ml

Add the following essential oils:
Atlas cedarwood 2 drops
Frankincense 7 drops
Geranium 4 drops
Lemon 5 drops
Rose 1 drop
Sweet orange 6 drops

Apply a moderate amount of the oil blend to your face, chest, and upper back at night time, and massage in well. Full details of how to give yourself a facial massage can be found in Chapter 6.

6.   ROSEHIP SEED OIL   Botanical name: *Rosa canina*

One of my favourite plant oils to use, and especially in pregnancy, is rosehip seed oil. In its organic form, it has a beautiful red tinge to its colour and has quite a distinctive smell. It is a luxurious oil that is beautifully balancing and highly restorative for the skin. Given that it is known as a dry, thin oil, the skin also quickly and easily absorbs it and it is excellent in helping with cell and tissue regeneration and for repairing strained or compromised skin. The good news is that it is wonderful in helping to overcome wrinkles, fine lines, and stretch marks. Rosehip seed oil has a very high content of polyunsaturated fatty acids, and can go rancid very easily. However, one way to ensure a longer shelf life of your oil is to buy it with vitamin E having been added as an anti-oxidant, and then to keep it in your fridge. Again, always remember to buy your oils in dark bottles, preferably glass, as this slows down any degradation by sunlight.

Regenerating Night Time Facial oil with Rosehip (30ml)

Rosehip oil 20ml
Grapeseed oil 5ml
Jojoba oil 5ml

<u>Add the following essential oils:</u>
Frankincense 2 drops
Lavender 3 drops
Rose 1 drop

Apply about 2ml of the oil blend to your face at night time, and massage in well. Full details of how to give yourself a facial massage can be found in Chapter 6.

CHAPTER 5

Hey, I didn't sign up for that! (Common pregnancy discomforts and aromatherapy blends to address them)

PREGNANCY IS ONE of the most amazing times in a woman's life. Amazing, because your body goes through so many dramatic changes, so quickly, automatically, and yet so perfectly. We don't have to think about what process we're going to carry out next, we don't have to tell the placenta to form, we don't have to tell the embryo to implant, we don't have to tell cells to split and start forming organs. All of this happens of its own accord once conception takes place.

For some women, the phenomenon of forty-two (or thereabouts) weeks of pregnancy comes and goes, ironically, without much ado. However, for some other women, there is a whole host of discomforts that accompany their changing shape and the process of growing their baby.

Here, I am going to outline and define some of these discomforts in which aromatherapy has been known to be of help and benefit.

Please note I am deliberately giving details of how many drops of essential oils to add to your blends. It is very important to follow these instructions, and even though it may seem that you are using very few drops, it will result in the correct, safe dosage for use in pregnancy.

Also, all of the aromatherapy blends listed below are safe for use in pregnancy, however they are not recommended for infants under three years of age.

1. ACHES AND PAINS (INCLUDING BACKACHE)

As our joints and ligaments stretch, and become looser and more flexible in pregnancy, it can mean that we suffer discomfort in these areas. Often we feel that our muscles are aching unlike they did before, with our legs feeling heavy and our back and shoulders holding tension and tiredness. Unsurprisingly, one of the most common complaints in pregnancy is back ache.

BACKACHE

Backache can be very common in pregnancy, not only because of your changing shape putting more pressure on your back as your belly moves forward but also because of pregnancy hormones like relaxin that act upon ligaments, making them looser and more flexible. Therefore, your pelvis is not as stable as it would normally be, and can result in an aching, tired back. Poor posture, or sitting in the same position for extended periods of time are also contributing factors if you are suffering from backache. Yoga and Pilates will help to maintain good posture and strengthen your core muscles, and reduce the discomfort in your back.

Suggested Essential Oils for Aches and Pains (Including backache)	Cubeb Frankincense Lavender Roman chamomile Rose Sandalwood Vetiver Ylang ylang
Blend	Use 50ml of your favourite carrier oil, and add the following: Cubeb 2 drop Lavender 4 drops Frankincense 4 drops Rose 1 drop Or Lavender 4 drops Roman chamomile 2 drops Sandalwood 1 drop Vetiver 1 drop Ylang ylang 1 drop
Bath	Add 10-15mls of your chosen blend to an already drawn, warm bath. Disperse the oil through the water, then get in and relax for about 20 minutes. Be extra careful getting into and out of the bath tub because the oil will make the surface very slippery.

Massage	Massage about 10ml of your blend all over your body, paying particular attention to your back, neck, shoulders, hips, and legs. You may need to ask a loved one to help you for the harder to reach areas.

2. ANXIETY

Anxiety can happen for any number of reasons, and pregnancy can bring forth a whole host of concerns for a woman even though she may not consider herself to be an anxious person in general. In fact, a woman might be feeling anxious simply because she is pregnant. Is my baby ok? How will I cope with a baby/another baby? How will the birth go? All of these fears contribute to a state of stress that inhibits the body from functioning at its optimum and may impinge on the baby's development.

Symptoms of anxiety may include fearfulness, sleeplessness, tearfulness, breathing difficulties and bouts of excessive perspiration. However, aromatherapy is truly wonderful in helping to address anxieties, and can help you to deal with potential daily upsets much more easily.

Suggested Essential Oils for Anxiety	Atlas cedarwood
	Bergamot
	Frankincense
	Lavender
	Mandarin
	Neroli
	Patchouli
	Roman chamomile
	Rose
	Vetiver
	Ylang ylang

Blend	Use 50ml of your preferred carrier oil and add the following: Atlas cedarwood 1 drop Bergamot 3 drops Lavender 3 drops Patchouli 1 drop Rose 1 drop Or Frankincense 4 drops Lavender 5 drops Rose 1 drop Vetiver 1 drop Or Mandarin 6 drops Neroli 2 drops Roman chamomile 2 drops Ylang ylang 1 drop
Massage	Use a moderate amount of your blend and massage it all over your body, or at least areas like your hands, arms, face, neck, and shoulders, and if you have someone to help, your back as well. Breathe deeply, and relax. Use long, slow, relaxing strokes to help calm and comfort.

Bath	Use 10-15mls of your chosen blend and add it to a warm, drawn bath. Disperse the oil with your hand, get in, and relax for about 20 minutes. Be very careful getting into and out of the bath tub as the oils will mean that the surface will become very slippery.
Inhalation	In acute instances of anxiety, inhaling essential oils from a tissue will help you to overcome the intense emotions or feelings of overwhelm. Use any of the following: Lavender 1 drop Neroli 1 drop Or Frankincense 1 drop Lavender 1 drop Or Roman chamomile 1 drop Rose 1 drop Or Lavender 1 drop Vetiver 1 drop

Vaporisation/Diffusion	Add the following to your oil burner or diffuser: Lavender 1 drop Mandarin 2 drops Neroli 1 drop Or Bergamot 2 drops Frankincense 1 drop Patchouli 1 drop Or Mandarin 3 drops Ylang ylang 1 drop

3. BREAST TENDERNESS

Often breast tenderness can be one of the initial signs of pregnancy for a woman. Even in the very first weeks, the body is undergoing such profound changes and the breasts are developing in preparation for breastfeeding. There is an increase in blood flow to breast tissue, and a rapid development of milk-producing cells, called acini, and milk ducts. This often leads to noticeable breast growth which can be accompanied by extreme sensitivity, heat, and for many women, tenderness in the area.

Suggested Essential Oils for Breast Tenderness	Geranium Lavender Mandarin Roman chamomile

Blend	Use 50ml of your preferred carrier oil and add the following: Geranium 2 drops Lavender 3 drops Mandarin 5 drops Roman chamomile 2 drops
Compress	Add 10mls of your blend to a bowl/basin of comfortably warm water and mix it through with your hand. Soak a face flannel in the oil/water, wring out, and then apply directly to the breast area. Leave on until the flannel loses its warmth. Rinse and repeat. You can do one breast at a time, or have two flannels and use them on both breasts at the same time. It may help to be lying down or in a semi-reclined position so that you can relax with the compress applied.
Bath	Add 10-15mls of your blend to an already drawn, warm bath. Disperse the oil through the water, then get in and relax for about 20 minutes. Be extra careful getting into and out of the bath tub because the oil will make the surface very slippery.

Massage (very gently)	Use a moderate amount of your blend and massage it *very gently* into your breasts. This will improve blood flow to the area. The essential oils will help to reduce the inflammation and the sense of heat that accompanies it.

4. BREATHLESSNESS

Breathlessness can be experienced early in your pregnancy, (in fact it was one of the first signs for me!) as well as later in the 42 weeks. At the beginning of pregnancy, breathlessness occurs due to the rapid pace at which the embryo is developing. Simply put, your blood system is having difficulty keeping up the oxygen supply that your growing baby is demanding. Therefore, you will breathe more frequently in an attempt to increase your oxygen supply. Later in pregnancy, you may experience breathlessness because your heart and lungs are working harder to provide oxygen all over your now bigger body and of course to your growing baby. There is also more pressure put on your lungs due to the increased size of your womb.

Essential oils that encourage deep, relaxed breathing may be of benefit here.

Suggested Essential Oils for Breathlessness	Atlas cedarwood Cubeb Frankincense Lavender Ylang ylang

Blend	Atlas cedarwood 1 drop Frankincense 1 drop Lavender 1 drop Or Atlas cedarwood 1 drop Cubeb 1 drop Ylang ylang 1 drop Please note that there is no need for a carrier oil here as the blends are only going to be used in a diffuser or oil burner.
Vaporiser	Vaporise one of the above blends in your diffuser or oil burner for about 30 minutes

5. CARPAL TUNNEL SYNDROME

When the nerves and tendons in your hands and wrists are subjected to increased pressure from the greater amount of fluid in your pregnant body, you may feel tingling, numbness or pain in your fingers, hands, and wrists that can radiate upwards into your arm. This pain and discomfort can be very debilitating, and can often be worse in the morning time upon waking. It is important to contact a chartered physiotherapist who can help you with supporting your arm and wrist. They will also be able to show you appropriate exercises to help lessen the discomfort somewhat. In aromatherapy terms, you may find similar essential oils that are helpful in treating oedema to be useful in the treatment of carpal tunnel syndrome. However, pain-relieving oils will also be a valuable addition to the blend.

Suggested Essential Oils for Carpal Tunnel Syndrome	Atlas cedarwood Cubeb Cypress Geranium Lavender Roman chamomile
Blend	Use 50ml of your preferred carrier oil and add the following: Atlas cedarwood 1 drop Cubeb 1 drop Cypress 2 drops Geranium 3 drops Lavender 3 drops Roman chamomile 2 drops
Massage	Use a moderate amount of your blend and massage it in gently to your hands, wrists, and forearms, in an upward motion. This will improve blood flow to the area, and help to remove excess fluid. The essential oils will help to reduce the inflammation, the swelling, and the pain that accompanies it.

Cold compress	Add 10mls of your blend to a bowl/basin of cool water and mix it through with your hand. Soak a face flannel in the oil-water blend, wring out, and then apply directly to the hands and wrists. Leave on for about 5 minutes on each hand. Rinse and repeat. You can do one hand at a time, or have two flannels and use them on both hands at the same time. It may help to be in a semi-reclined or seated position so that you can relax with the compress applied.
Bath	Add 10-15mls of your blend to an already drawn, warm bath. Disperse the oil through the water, then get in and relax for about 20 minutes. Be extra careful getting into and out of the bath tub because the oil will make the surface very slippery.

6. COLD SORES

The appearance of a cold sore can more than ruin not only your day but indeed your week! If you have ever had a cold sore, the herpes simplex virus that causes them more often than not lies dormant within your system. However, when a woman is pregnant, her immune system may at times become compromised because her body is directing so much of its energies towards growing and protecting her baby. Unfortunately, an unsightly cold sore can erupt. Furthermore, it is critical that you do not kiss your baby on the face if you have a cold sore when the child is born, as the herpes simplex virus can be extremely dangerous for a baby.

Most over the counter cold sore remedies are not recommended when a woman is pregnant, so essential oils offer a safe and effective answer to the problem.

Suggested Essential Oils for Cold Sores	Bergamot, Geranium** Lemon (**I have found geranium to be particularly effective)
Blend	10ml Grapeseed oil Geranium 3 drops Or Bergamot 1 drop Geranium 1 drop Lemon 1 drop
Application	Using a clean cotton bud, apply some of the blend to the area of the tingle, or cold sore itself if it has already erupted. Repeat up to 3 times daily. Keep it away from the inner lips and cheek. Do not swallow.

7. CONSTIPATION

The rise in the level of the hormone progesterone in pregnancy causes your intestines to relax and become more sluggish. This can lead to constipation, which is often exacerbated if a woman is taking iron supplements while pregnant.

Constipation should not be overlooked, or ignored as it can be very uncomfortable and may lead to other conditions like haemorrhoids, headaches, general sluggishness, backache, and oedema. In severe cases, being constipated can negatively impact on so many other aspects of your life such as your mood, ability to walk comfortably, and overall emotional well-being. None of which, as I am sure you will agree, is any fun.

Eating plenty of fresh produce, reducing processed foods, increasing your intake of water, and reducing your consumption of caffeine will obviously help with keeping your digestive system working as it should. Also, exercise like walking, swimming, yoga or Pilates can assist in keeping things moving.

Essential oils that can improve the discomfort of constipation are ones that are cleansing, and that can stimulate the bowels. If there is an emotional aspect to a woman being constipated, for example fear, or stress, then essential oils which address these emotions can be used. It may be advisable to go and have a treatment with a trained aromatherapist to have a personalised blend of essential oils made for you to address specific emotional factors. Reflexology is also an excellent way to help alleviate the discomforts of constipation, and hand reflexology is something that you can use on yourself anytime, anywhere. It is a good idea to visit a reflexologist for treatment, however, you can work on your own hands at home. Please go to www.AromaBump.com to see a video of how to do this.

Suggested Essential Oils for Constipation	Cardamom Ginger Grapefruit Lemon Sweet orange Peppermint

Blend	Use 50ml of your preferred carrier oil and add the following: Sweet orange 5 drops Peppermint 1 drop Ginger 2 drop, Grapefruit 4 drops Or Cardamom 3 drops Sweet orange 7 drops Peppermint 1 drop
Massage	Massage a moderate amount of the blend slowly into your abdomen, in a clockwise direction as you look down at your belly. Continue this for three to four minutes. It would also be helpful if a loved one massaged your lower back in the same manner.
Bath	Add 10-15mls of your blend to an already drawn, warm bath. Disperse the oil through the water, then get in and relax for about 20 minutes. Be extra careful getting into and out of the bath tub because the oil will make the surface very slippery.

8. CYSTITIS & URINARY TRACT INFECTIONS (UTIs)

Cystitis is inflammation of the bladder due to a bacterial infection, and this and other urinary tract infections (UTIs) can often plague a woman during her pregnancy. Given that our body is experiencing an increase in the hormone relaxin, our tubes carrying urine away from the bladder, the ureters, can kink and curve a bit like a hosepipe. Bacteria can easily become trapped in these little bends and result in a bladder infection. Sometimes these infections have no symptoms whatsoever other than the appearance of leukocytes or blood in the urine. However, it is important to address them. My own opinion is that it is better for your body and your baby to avoid the use of antibiotics during pregnancy as many other options work in a kinder way with your body. However, sometimes it may be necessary to take antibiotics if the infection is particularly severe or persistent. Diet is also a major factor in improving your overall immunity and wellbeing.

From personal experience, I also found the use of reflexology and acupuncture in pregnancy to be wonderfully beneficial in overcoming UTIs, but it is important to consult your primary caregiver in this matter.

Suggested Essential Oils for Cystitis & UTIs	Bergamot Cubeb Fragonia Lavender Lemon Sandalwood
Blend	Use 50ml of your preferred carrier oil and add the following: Bergamot 3 drops Fragonia 4 drops Lavender 3 drops Sandalwood 2 drops Or Cubeb 3 drops Lavender 4 drops Lemon 5 drops

Bath	Add 10-15mls of your chosen blend to an already drawn, warm bath. Disperse the oil through the water, then get in and relax for about 20 minutes. Be extra careful getting into and out of the bath tub because the oil will make the surface very slippery.
Massage	Massage a moderate amount of the blend slowly into your lower abdomen, in a clockwise direction as you look down at your belly. Continue this for three to four minutes. It would also be helpful if a loved one massaged your back in the same manner.
Sitz Bath	**Adjust your blend to the following:** 50 ml carrier oil Bergamot 1 drop Fragonia 2 drops Lavender 1 drop Sandalwood 1 drop Fill your Sitz bath appropriately with warm water and disperse 10mls of your blend through the water. Sit and relax for 5 minutes with your bottom resting in the warm water.

9. DEPRESSION

We often hear about someone suffering from postnatal depression, however depression before baby is born is also common, yet not often acknowledged, or talked about. First and foremost with any sort of mental health, it is very important to talk about how you are feeling with a loved one, or perhaps a friend who may have experienced something similar in her pregnancy, your GP, or midwife. Don't feel that you are by yourself in this situation even if you are feeling overwhelmed by the reality of your pregnancy, or that it was unexpected or even unwanted.

Aromatherapy can be very supportive in times like these, and many essential oils can be used.

Suggested essential oils for Depression	Atlas cedarwood
	Bergamot
	Fragonia
	Frankincense
	Geranium
	Grapefruit
	Lemon
	Mandarin
	Neroli
	Patchouli
	Roman chamomile
	Rose
	Sweet orange

Blend	Use 50ml of your preferred carrier oil and add the following: Bergamot 4 drops Geranium 2 drops Patchouli 1 drop Sweet orange 5 drops Or Atlas cedarwood 1 drop Grapefruit 4 drops Frankincense 2 drops Mandarin 4 drops Neroli 1 drop Or Fragonia 5 drops Lavender 3 drops Patchouli 1 drop Rose 1 drop There are many wonderful blending options given that there are so many essential oils that are useful for helping with depression. You might like to come up with your own blends once you follow the blending guidelines detailed in the essential oil profiles in chapter 3.

Bath	Add 10-15mls of your blend to an already drawn, warm bath. Disperse the oil through the water, then get in and relax for about 20 minutes. Be extra careful getting into and out of the bath tub because the oil will make the surface very slippery.
Massage	Massage a moderate amount of your chosen blend all over your body, paying particular attention to your upper body, neck, back, and head.
Vaporisation	The following blends can be used in your oil burner or diffuser. Use for about 30 minutes, stop, then resume after about an hour for another 30 minutes. Atlas cedarwood 1 drop Grapefruit 1 drop Mandarin 2 drops Or Geranium 1 drop Fragonia 1 drop Frankincense 1 drop Sweet orange 1 drop Or Lemon 2 drops Sweet orange 1 drop Atlas cedarwood 1 drop

10. HAEMORRHOIDS & VULVAL VARICOSITIES

Haemorrhoids are varicose veins that happen in and around the anus. They are extremely uncomfortable, itchy, and painful. Do everything in your power to avoid getting them in the first place (drink lots of water, reduce caffeine, eat lots of fresh fruit and vegetables, reduce sugar and salt, and keep active). In pregnancy, they can occur due to the increase in weight on your pelvic floor, and if you're constipated and have to strain to empty your bowels, then you have to put more pressure on your rectum and pelvic floor. They can also happen if you go through prolonged pushing during your labour and birth.

Vulval varicosities are similar to haemorrhoids except for the fact that they occur in your vulva or lower vagina. These are also extremely uncomfortable and can cause severe discomfort and itching. They occur, once again, as a result of the increased pressure on your pelvic floor, and the increased pressure on the blood vessels in and around the vulva and vaginal wall.

Essential oils can help to reduce the haemorrhoids in size, and help to heal them if they tear when passing stools. They will also ease the discomfort of vulval varicosities in a similar way.

Suggested Essential Oils for Haemorrhoids and/or Vulval Varicosities	Cypress Geranium Grapefruit Lemon
Blend	Use 50ml of your preferred carrier oil and add the following: Cypress 2 drops Geranium 2 drops Grapefruit 4 drops Lemon 4 drops

Bath	Add 10-15mls of your blend to an already drawn, warm bath. Disperse the oil through the water, then get in and relax for about 20 minutes. Be extra careful getting into and out of the bath tub because the oil will make the surface very slippery.
Sitz Bath	**Adjust your blend to the following:** 50 ml carrier oil Cypress 1 drop Geranium 1 drop Grapefruit 1 drop Lemon 1 drop Fill your Sitz bath appropriately with warm water and disperse 10mls of your blend through the water. Sit and relax for 5 minutes with your bottom resting in the warm water.

11. HAYFEVER

Having hayfever is normally bad enough. However, couple it with being pregnant and not being able to take any over the counter remedies with anti-histamine, and it can equal a not-very-pleasant experience. The symptoms of streaming eyes and nose, blocked sinuses, itchy throat, and headache can prove very uncomfortable for a pregnant woman. Once again, while not curing the problem, aromatherapy can help to alleviate some of the discomforts.

Suggested Essential Oils for Hayfever	Atlas cedarwood Cypress Eucalyptus Frankincense Lavender Lemon Roman chamomile Rose
Blend	Use 50ml of grapeseed oil and add the following: Atlas cedarwood 2 drops Cypress 2 drops Lemon 5 drops Eucalyptus 2 drops Or Atlas cedarwood 2 drops Frankincense 3 drops Lavender 3 drops Roman chamomile 2 drops Rose 1 drop
Facial massage	Apply about 5ml of your blend to your face, neck, and chest, and massage in well. Please refer to Chapter 6 for full details on how to carry out a facial massage

Steam inhalation	Add the following to a facial sauna, or simply a (ceramic or metal) bowl of warm water and placing your head close, inhale for about 10 minutes:
	Atlas cedarwood 1 drop Eucalyptus 1 drop
	Or Lavender 1 drop Lemon 1 drop
	Or Eucalyptus 1 drop Frankincense 1 drop
	If you find that the steam and/or essential oils are too strong when inhaling, move your face back a little from the facial sauna or bowl of warm water. Take regular short breaks during the process.
Vaporisation	Add the following to your oil burner or plug-in diffuser and leave it on for 30 minutes: Lavender 1 drop Lemon 2 drops Eucalyptus 1 drop
	Or Atlas cedarwood 1 drop Roman chamomile 1 drop Lavender 2 drops

12. HEADACHES

Headaches can be quite common both in early pregnancy as well as further along. They can be caused by hormonal changes, sensitivities to smells, stress, tension, tiredness or dehydration.

The first thing I recommend, perhaps unsurprisingly, is to drink more water and to get some fresh air, as often headaches are exacerbated by being inside in a stuffy environment. This can happen so easily if you're working in a shared workplace, or in an area with poor ventilation.

In terms of aromatherapy, lavender is my first port of call for alleviating headaches. With its wonderfully sweet, herbaceous aroma, it blends beautifully with so many other essential oils, including geranium and roman chamomile.

I should point out, however, that when used in excess, lavender can have the opposite effect to the desired one. For example, when used excessively, instead of alleviating a headache, it can encourage one; instead of helping with insomnia, too much lavender can keep you awake.

This is just one example of why using the correct amounts and dilutions is so important.

Suggested Essential Oils for Headaches	Geranium
	Lavender
	Lemon
	Mandarin
	Roman chamomile

Vaporiser/Diffuser	Add the following to your vaporiser/diffuser: Lavender 1 drop Lemon 1 drop Or Lemon 1 drop Mandarin 1 drop Or Mandarin 1 drop Roman chamomile 1 drop Or Lemon 1 drop Geranium 1 drop
Room spray	Mist a few sprays of lavender floral water around your room
Facial/Head massage	Use 50ml of your preferred carrier oil and add the following: Geranium 1 drop Lavender 2 drops Lemon 2 drops Roman chamomile 1 drop Massage a moderate amount all over your face, up the back of your neck and through your hair. For full instructions on how to carry out a facial massage, please refer to Chapter 6.

Bath (especially if you have a tension headache)	Add 10-15mls of your blend to an already drawn, warm bath. Disperse the oil through the water, then get in and relax for about 20 minutes. Be extra careful getting into and out of the bath tub because the oil will make the surface very slippery.

13. HEARTBURN

Once again we point to the relaxing effects of pregnancy hormones on smooth muscle as being the culprit for another discomfort; heartburn. A woman, even early in her pregnancy, can be affected by the discomfort of heartburn, but it is more prevalent in the third trimester when her bump is larger and is pressing upwards on her stomach and diaphragm. The little sphincter muscle which normally keeps the stomach acid tightly enclosed within the stomach sac tends to relax a little in pregnancy and does not do its job quite as efficiently as normal. Therefore, some stomach acid is able to escape upwards towards the oesophagus causing the uncomfortable burning sensation which is commonly referred to as heartburn.

Stress may make heartburn worse, as may certain foods, and I definitely recommend reflexology and acupuncture to help alleviate this discomfort, but aromatherapy can also be of some benefit.

Suggested Essential Oils for Heartburn	Cardamom Grapefruit Peppermint Roman chamomile Sweet orange

Blend	Use 50ml of your preferred carrier oil and add the following: Cardamom 2 drops Grapefruit 4 drops Peppermint 1 drop Roman chamomile 2 drops Sweet orange 3 drops
Massage	Using gentle massage apply a moderate amount of your blend over the top of your bump, under and between your breasts and over your chest and back.
Bath	Add 10-15mls of your blend to an already drawn, warm bath. Disperse the oil through the water, then get in and relax for about 20 minutes. Be extra careful getting into and out of the bath tub because the oil will make the surface very slippery.

14. HIPS

In pregnancy, as baby develops and grows bigger, our poor hips can be subjected to so much pressure that it can cause major discomfort, tiredness, and pain; sometimes you might even feel like your hips are going to break apart! It can also be a real problem at night time, when we're told to lie on our left side, but then it gets too painful and we have to keep changing sides, which leads to much disrupted and uncomfortable sleep.

Massage and warm baths are probably the best ways to improve the discomfort of painful hips and essential oils that are analgesic or are topical circulatory stimulants (TCS), in that they encourage greater blood flow to the area, will be the most beneficial.

Suggested Essential Oils for Sore Hips	Cubeb Frankincense Lavender Roman chamomile Vetiver Ylang ylang
Blend	Use 50ml of your preferred carrier oil and add the following: Cubeb 2 drops Frankincense 3 drops Lavender 3 drops Roman Chamomile 2 drops Vetiver 1 drop Ylang ylang 1 drop
Massage	Use a moderate amount of your blend and massage it well into your lower back, hips, buttocks, and upper thighs. Be careful not to apply too much pressure to your sacrum area before full term pregnancy.
Bath	Use 10-15mls of your blend and add it to a warm, drawn bath. Disperse the oil with your hand, get in, and relax for about 20 minutes. Be careful getting in and out of the bath tub as the oils will cause the surface to become slippery.

15. HYPERTENSION (High Blood Pressure)

Hypertension or high blood pressure is an extremely common condition encountered during pregnancy, complicating around 2-3% of pregnancies and a slight rise in BP is often only a normal characteristic of a woman's pregnant body. Stress and tension can affect a woman's blood pressure and it is this aspect that can be addressed with aromatherapy.

However, please note that raised blood pressure in pregnancy, which can be normal for the most part, can also be a sign of preeclampsia especially if accompanied by protein in your urine sample, persistent or dramatic swelling in legs, feet and hands or face, headaches, and palpitations. Therefore, please be vigilant about contacting your caregiver immediately if you experience any of these symptoms.

If, however, your raised blood pressure is simply due to your body changing in pregnancy, and the extra volume of blood that that entails and nothing untoward, then using essential oils can really improve the situation.

Suggested essential oils for Hypertension	Frankincense
	Lavender
	Neroli
	Roman chamomile
	Rose
	Sandalwood
	Vetiver
	Ylang ylang

Blend	Use 50ml of your preferred carrier oil and add the following: Frankincense 4 drops Lavender 4 drops Roman chamomile 2 drops Sandalwood 2 drops Or Lavender 4 drops Neroli 2 drops Rose 1 drop Ylang ylang 1 drop Or Frankincense 4 drops Lavender 4 drops Rose 1 drop Vetiver 1 drop
Bath	Use 10-15mls of your chosen blend and add it to a warm, drawn bath. Disperse the oil with your hand, get in, and relax for about 20 minutes. Be careful getting in and out of the bath tub as the oils will cause the surface to become slippery.
Massage	Use a moderate amount of your blend and massage it all over your body, or at least areas like your hands, arms, face, neck, and shoulders and if you have someone to help, your back as well. Breathe deeply, and relax.

Vaporisation/Diffusion	Use either of the following blends in your oil burner or diffuser for 30 minutes: Frankincense 1 drop Lavender 1 drop Roman chamomile 1 drop Or Lavender 1 drop Neroli 1 drop Ylang ylang 1 drop
Inhalation	In acute cases of (non-preeclampsia related) raised blood pressure, e.g. when in a hospital or visiting your GP and you experience White Coat Syndrome, inhalation of essential oils from a tissue can help. Frankincense 1 drop Or Rose 1 drop Or Ylang ylang 1 drop Or Lavender 1 drop Or Sandalwood 1 drop

16. MORNING SICKNESS/NAUSEA

Morning sickness can be a bit of a misnomer because unfortunately for some women, it can last all day, for as long as 16 weeks, and for the very unfortunate ones, right through their pregnancy.

The nausea that we refer to as morning sickness can occur as a result of sharp changes in hormones, low blood sugars, or tiredness, and can manifest as straightforward nausea, or may be accompanied by vomiting. Either way, it's not a pleasant condition.

For some women, eating small, but frequent snacks like dry crackers or something like a digestive biscuit, especially first thing in the morning has been known to help. I am also aware, anecdotally, that chewing on raw almonds can also relieve the discomfort. Drinking teas like chamomile, peppermint or ginger might also quash the queasiness.

Essential oils like peppermint, lemon, ginger or cardamom may be helpful in alleviating the uncomfortable sensation of nausea for some women.

Suggested Essential Oils for Morning Sickness	Cardamom Ginger Lemon Peppermint Sweet orange
Blend	Use 50ml of your preferred carrier oil and add the following: Cardamom 2 drops Ginger 2 drops Lemon 4 drops Peppermint 1 drop Sweet orange 3 drops
Bath	Use 10-15mls of your chosen blend and add it to a warm, drawn bath. Disperse the oil with your hand, get in, and relax for about 20 minutes. Be careful getting in and out of the bath tub as the oils will cause the surface to become slippery.

Massage	Massage a moderate amount of your blend into hands, neck, upper chest, and scalp for about 5 minutes.
Vaporisation	Add the following to your oil burner or diffuser for 30 minutes: Cardamom 1 drop Ginger 1 drop Lemon 2 drops Or Lemon 2 drops Peppermint 1 drop Sweet orange 1 drop

17. OEDEMA

During your pregnancy, after being on your feet for a long time, wearing restrictive clothing, or in warm weather, many women experience swelling, or oedema in their feet, ankles, legs, and hands. This can be very uncomfortable, and in some instances, can prove quite serious as it can be a sign of preeclampsia. However, some accumulation of fluid is normal for many women and is merely a result of expanding blood vessels near the skin, which results in a greater amount of fluid in the tissues. Poor circulation and the weight of the uterus on the pelvic floor can mean that the lymphatic system has a harder time draining away excess fluid, so it is important to stay active during pregnancy, while still getting proper rest

Resting, and raising your ankles above your hips can help drain away some of the fluid, as can therapies like reflexology and acupuncture. Furthermore, massaging the areas prone to swelling, on a daily basis will help to keep it under control. The lymphatic system, which works to keep the body at normal fluid levels, does not have a pump of its own, so it must rely on the action of muscles that contract around the lymph vessels to help move the fluid along, and back towards the heart. This is why movement and exercise is so important.

Suggested Essential Oils for Oedema	Atlas cedarwood Cypress Geranium Grapefruit Lemon Mandarin
Blend	Use 50ml of your preferred carrier oil and add the following: Atlas cedarwood 1 drop Cypress 2 drops Geranium 2 drops Grapefruit 5 drops Or Atlas cedarwood 1 drop Cypress 1 drop Lemon 4 drops Mandarin 5 drops
Massage	Using a moderate amount of your chosen blend, apply firm, yet comfortable pressure and start massaging your feet upwards towards your ankle and lower leg. Always work towards your heart. If bending to reach your legs is uncomfortable or simply too optimistic, then ask another kind and obliging person to help you. You can also massage your hands, wrists, and arms in a similar fashion, as this will also encourage whole body circulation.

Bath	Use 10-15mls of your chosen blend and add it to a (not too) warm, drawn bath. Disperse the oil with your hand, get in, and relax for about 20 minutes. Be careful getting in and out of the bath tub as the oils will cause the surface to become slippery.
Compress	Add 10mls of your blend to a bowl/basin of lukewarm/cool water and mix it through with your hand. Soak a face flannel in the oil-water mixture, wring out, and then apply directly to your feet and ankles. Leave on for three or four minutes. Rinse and repeat. You can do one foot at a time, or have two flannels and use them on both feet at the same time. It may help to be lying down with your feet raised slightly so that you can relax and enjoy the feeling of the compress.

18. PERINEUM PREPARATION

The perineum is the area between the vagina and the rectum, and one that is prepared and ready to stretch easily over a baby's crowning head is indeed a happy one. It may not be an overly comfortable or easy thing to achieve, but partaking of perineal massage is extremely beneficial and worthwhile in preparing for labour and birth.

Essential Oils to help with Perineal Massage	Lavender Sandalwood
Blend	Sweet almond oil 30ml Jojoba oil 10ml Evening Primrose oil 5ml Wheatgerm oil 5ml Lavender 1 drop Sandalwood 1 drop
Massage	Sitting comfortably in a semi-propped up position with your knees bent towards you, hook your thumbs about an inch into the bottom of your vagina, with your fingers on your buttocks, and massage with a downward pulling action with your thumbs and forefingers, working towards your anus. Start off slowly and gently, taking long, slow, deep breaths to help you relax. It may feel a little uncomfortable or stingy at first, but as the skin gains in elasticity, and the muscles become more accustomed to being stretched, it becomes easier and more comfortable. Build up to about 10 minutes daily and perhaps work it into your bedtime routine. This can be carried out from around 34 weeks of pregnancy.

19.   RESTLESS LEGS

Restless leg syndrome occurs in 5 to 10 percent of the general population, but in 10 to 20 percent of pregnant women[7], and it is suggested that it may be related to iron deficiency anaemia and also magnesium deficiency. It follows therefore, that the first place to look in order to help with restless legs in pregnancy, is diet. Foods rich in easily absorbable iron include red meat, sardines, beans, lentils, broccoli, spinach, egg yolks, can be incorporated into the diet, and foods that inhibit iron absorption can be limited, or at least consumed at different times than the iron-rich foods. Sources of magnesium also include green leafy vegetables like kale, collard greens, nuts and seeds, avocados, bananas, and good news - dark chocolate!

In addition to an iron and magnesium rich diet, aromatherapy can help to alleviate the discomfort and annoyance associated with restless legs, and works wonders when combined with magnesium-laden Epsom salts in the bath.

Essential Oils to help with Restless Legs	Atlas cedarwood
	Frankincense
	Lavender
	Lemon
	Peppermint
	Vetiver

---

[7] Prof. Claudio Bassetti, Neurocentro della Svizzera Italiana in Lugano http://www.medicalnewstoday.com/releases/226951.php

Blend	Use 50ml of grapeseed oil and add the following: Atlas cedarwood 1 drop Lavender 4 drops Lemon 4 drops Frankincense 2 drops Or Lavender 4 drops Frankincense 3 drops Peppermint 1 drop Vetiver 1 drop
Bath	Add 15ml of your chosen blend into 1 cup/225g of Epsom salts. Mix thoroughly and then add to your already drawn, warm bath. Get in and relax for about 20 minutes. Be careful getting in and out of the bath tub as the oils will cause the surface to become slippery.
Massage	Using a moderate amount of your chosen blend, apply firm, yet comfortable pressure to your feet and legs and start massaging them upwards. Always work towards your heart. Massaging other areas of your body as well will encourage an improvement in your overall circulation.

Compress	Add 20mls of your blend to a basin of cool water and mix it through with your hand. Soak a hand towel in the oil/water, wring out, and then apply directly to your legs. Leave on for about 5 minutes on each leg. Rinse and repeat. You can do one leg at a time, or have two towels and use them on both legs at the same time. It may help to be in a semi-reclined position with your legs slightly raised so that you can relax with the compress applied.

20. SINUSES (Blocked, and also Sinus infection)

During pregnancy, women can be more prone to suffering from blocked sinuses, or if an infection sets in, sinusitis. For some women, it only occurs on one side of their face and it can be uncomfortable at best, and very painful at worst. Inflammation occurs in the mucous membranes of the sinuses and nasal cavities resulting in the sensation of being 'blocked up' or, alternatively, having a slightly runny nose. If you have sinusitis, you can expect greater amounts of thick, nasal mucus, which can vary in colour from green to dark orange. This increased volume of mucus puts pressure on facial cavities causing pain above and below the eyes, along the cheekbones and down the sides of the nose. Many over the counter remedies for sinus pain cannot be used in pregnancy due to their anti-histamine content.

Aromatherapy can be wonderful at easing the pressure in your face, and can also boost your immune system.

Suggested Essential Oils to use for help with Sinuses	Cardamom Cubeb Eucalyptus Lemon Lavender Peppermint Sandalwood
Blend	Use 50ml of grapeseed oil and add the following: Cubeb 2 drops Eucalyptus 2 drops Lemon 3 drops Lavender 3 drops Or Cardamom 2 drops Lemon 4 drops Peppermint 1 drop Sandalwood 1 drop
Facial massage	Massage a moderate amount of your blend all over your face and neck, paying particular attention to the areas across your forehead, eyebrows, under the bony area of your eye sockets, and under your cheekbones; always working from the centre of your face, out towards your ears. For a full description of a facial massage, please refer to Chapter 6.

Inhalation	Add the following to a facial sauna, or simply a (ceramic or metal) bowl of warm water for about 10 minutes and inhale: Cubeb 1 drop Eucalyptus 1 drop Or Lavender 1 drop Lemon 1 drop Or Peppermint 1 drop Sandalwood 1 drop If you notice that the steam and/or essential oils are too strong when inhaling, move your face back a little from the facial sauna or bowl of warm water. Take regular short breaks during the process.

Vaporisation	Add any of the following blends to your oil burner or diffuser and use in a room for about 30 minutes. Turn off for an hour and resume for another 30 minutes. Cubeb 1 drop Eucalyptus 1 drop Lemon 1 drop Or Peppermint 1 drop Lavender 1 drop Lemon 1 drop

21. SLEEPLESSNESS

Ironically, despite the tiredness that you can experience in pregnancy, many women suffer from insomnia, be it difficulty in falling asleep due to discomfort, or waking up in the middle of the night to use the bathroom and not being able to get back to sleep again. All of this can be very frustrating, and depleting, especially if you have to get up to go to work, or be alert and fit to look after other children the following day and will have no opportunity for a nap.

Some essential oils are wonderfully sleep-inducing and this soporific quality makes them perfect for evening time use.

Suggested Essential Oils for Sleeplessness	Frankincense Geranium Lavender Neroli Roman chamomile Rose Sandalwood Vetiver Ylang ylang
Blend	Use 50ml of your preferred carrier oil and add the following: Frankincense 3 drops Lavender 4 drops Roman chamomile 2 drops Rose 1 drop Or Geranium 1 drop Lavender 3 drops Neroli 2 drops Sandalwood 1 drop Ylang ylang 1 drop Or Frankincense 4 drops Lavender 4 drops Rose 1 drop Vetiver 1 drop

Bath	For evening time: Use 10-15mls of your chosen blend and add it to a warm, drawn bath. Disperse the oil with your hand, get in and relax for about 20 minutes. Be careful getting in and out of the tub as the oils will cause the surface to become slippery.
Massage	As part of your night time routine, use a moderate amount of your chosen blend and massage all over your body. If you're at the stage of your pregnancy where you can't reach much of your body easily, simply focus on massaging your hands, arms, chest, neck, and face before going to bed.
Vaporisation/Diffusion	Drop the following blend onto a tissue and place it over a warm radiator in your bedroom as you get ready for bed, or place it on your bedside table if the radiators are not on. Frankincense 1 drop Geranium 1 drop Lavender 1 drop Roman chamomile 1 drop

22. STRESS

Stress can wreak havoc in anyone's life, and in pregnancy it is no different. In simple terms, if you are stressed, your body is in fight or flight mode and not functioning as it should – not paying attention to the non-essential functions for survival. (Unfortunately, growing a baby is not seen as a survival absolute when you're meant to be fleeing immediate danger.) Of course we all need some level of stress in our lives to motivate us and propel us to do things on a daily basis, but if stress is allowed to take hold and we end up living in a stressed environment and stressed body, a pregnant woman will pass these stress hormones on to her baby. Stress in pregnancy will constrict the blood vessels leading to your womb and will reduce the level of oxygen and nutrients reaching your baby. If you are stressed, your immune system will be compromised and you are more likely to succumb to sickness and fatigue.

Aromatherapy is truly wonderful in helping to alleviate stress and improve the body's functioning and to help you deal with daily stresses much more easily.

Suggested Essential Oils for Stress	Atlas cedarwood Bergamot Frankincense Lavender Mandarin Nerol Patchouli Roman chamomile Rose Vetiver Ylang ylang

Blend	Use 50ml of your preferred carrier oil and add the following: Atlas cedarwood 1 drop Bergamot 3 drops Lavender 3 drops Patchouli 1 drop Rose 1 drop Or Frankincense 4 drops Lavender 5 drops Rose 1 drop Vetiver 1 drop Or Mandarin 6 drops Neroli 2 drops Roman chamomile 2 drops Ylang ylang 1 drop
Massage	Use a moderate amount of your blend and massage it in all over your body, or at least areas like your hands and arms, face, neck and shoulders and if you have someone to help, your back as well. Breathe deeply, and relax. Use long, slow, relaxing strokes to help calm and comfort.
Bath	Use 10-15mls of your chosen blend and add it to a warm, drawn bath. Disperse the oil with your hand, and get in and relax for about 20 minutes.

Inhalation	In acute instances of stress, inhaling essential oils from a tissue will help you to overcome the intense emotions or feelings of overwhelm. Use any of the following: Lavender 1 drop Neroli 1 drop Or Frankincense 1 drop Lavender 1 drop Or Roman chamomile 1 drop Rose 1 drop Or Lavender 1 drop Vetiver 1 drop
Vaporisation/Diffusion	Add the following to your oil burner or diffuser: Lavender 1 drop Mandarin 2 drops Neroli 1 drop Or Bergamot 2 drops Frankincense 1 drop Patchouli 1 drop Or Mandarin 3 drops Ylang ylang 1 drop

23. SYMPHYSIS PUBIS DYSFUNCTION (SPD)

Symphysis Pubis Dysfunction, or SPD, is when the bones of the pelvis become unstable due to the effect of pregnancy hormones. The cartilage holding the pubic bone in its secure position becomes softer and great discomfort is caused when a pregnant woman walks, raises her leg to walk up stairs or when she moves her leg in a sideways motion, as if to get into a car. Many women having seen their ante-natal physiotherapist are recommended to use crutches and pelvic support belts which reduce the level of pelvic mobility.

While aromatherapy will not cure the cause of SPD, it may be used to ease the discomfort and relieve the stress that the body is holding in the affected muscle groups.

Suggested Essential Oils for SPD	Frankincense Lavender Roman chamomile Rose Vetiver
Blend	Use 50ml of your preferred carrier oil and add the following: Frankincense 3 drops Lavender 4 drops Roman chamomile 3 drops Rose 1 drop Vetiver 1 drop
Massage	Use a moderate amount of your blend and massage it well into your lower back, hips, buttocks, upper thighs, lower abdomen, and pubic bone. Be careful not to apply too much pressure to your sacrum area before full term pregnancy.

Bath	Use 10-15mls of your chosen blend and add it to a warm, drawn bath. Disperse the oil with your hand, get in, and relax for about 20 minutes. **As always, but especially so in the case of SPD, USE EXTREME CAUTION GETTING INTO AND OUT OF THE BATH TUB – ALWAYS HAVE SOMEONE ELSE TO HELP YOU** as the oils will cause the surface to become slippery.

24.   STRETCH MARKS - See Chapter 6 "Your Pregnancy Skin."

25.   THRUSH

The occurrence of thrush in pregnancy is quite common, given the change in acidity of a woman's vagina and vulva. It can also happen as a result of taking antibiotics because these kill off the good bacteria as well as the bad bacteria in your gut, affecting the proper balance of your internal flora. The symptoms include having a heavy, itchy, sometimes bad-smelling vaginal discharge, and/or a swollen and inflamed vulva. It is exceedingly uncomfortable and can seem to affect your whole being and sense of wellness. There may also be emotional aspects at play, especially if a woman is fearful during her pregnancy or perhaps unwelcoming of her changing shape, or feeling vulnerable.

Suggested Essential Oils for Thrush	Bergamot Fragonia Lavender Sandalwood

Blend	Use 50ml of your preferred carrier oil and add the following: Bergamot 2 drops Fragonia 3 drops Lavender 3 drops Sandalwood 2 drops
Bath	Use 10-15mls of your blend and add it to a warm, drawn bath. Disperse the oil with your hand, get in, and relax for about 20 minutes. Remember to be extra careful getting into and out of the bath tub due to the oils making the surface slippery.
Compress	Add 10mls of your blend to a bowl/basin of cool water and mix it through with your hand. Soak a face flannel in the oil-water mixture, wring out, and then apply directly to your vulva and perineum, being careful to avoid direct contact with the anal area. Keep pressed to the area for three or four minutes. Rinse and repeat. You may find it more comfortable to be in a semi-reclining position on your bed with a towel underneath you.

Sitz bath	**Adjust your blend to the following**: 50ml of your preferred carrier oil Bergamot 1 drop Fragonia 1 drop Lavender 2 drops Sandalwood 1 drop Fill your Sitz bath appropriately with warm water and disperse 10mls of your blend through the water. Sit and relax for 5 minutes with your bottom resting in the warm water.
Natural yogurt	Using 50ml of full-fat natural yogurt add your essential oils and mix thoroughly: Bergamot 1 drop Fragonia 1 drop Lavender 2 drops Sandalwood 1 drop Apply about 10ml directly in and around your vulva area, but do not insert it into your vagina. This can be left on, and reapplied twice more throughout the day. Wearing a panty liner will protect your underwear. Keep the remaining yogurt blend in the fridge in an airtight container (preferably glass or ceramic), and label it accordingly.

26. TIREDNESS

Probably one of the first symptoms a woman can experience in pregnancy is extreme tiredness. That sensation of hitting an invisible wall, of trying to drag your legs through what feels like wallpaper paste as you walk, accompanied by the immense yawns that overtake you. The body is undergoing the greatest changes that it will ever know in the first few weeks of pregnancy and all of your energy is directed towards your baby's exponential growth. This can leave you feeling depleted, exhausted, and simply unable to keep going.

Here we have two options with aromatherapy: Use essential oils to help overcome the tiredness and assist in sustaining your energy, or use oils that work hand in hand with your tiredness and promote deep, beneficial sleep and rest.

My first advice is; if you can nap, then do so — nothing feels quite so wonderful, and rest is of utmost importance. However, if it's during the daytime and you're at work, minding other children, or are otherwise occupied and you have no opportunity to sleep, then it would be beneficial to use uplifting, energising oils.

Suggested Essential Oils for Tiredness	To sustain energy levels: Bergamot Cubeb Grapefruit Lemon Sweet orange To encourage sleep: Frankincense Lavender Roman chamomile Sandalwood Ylang ylang

Blend	Use 50ml of your preferred carrier oil and add the following: (Sustain energy levels) Bergamot 2 drops Cubeb 2 drops Grapefruit 2 drops Lemon 4 drops Sweet orange 2 drops (Encourage Sleep) Frankincense 3 drops Lavender 4 drops Roman chamomile 2 drops Sandalwood 1 drop Ylang ylang 1 drop
Massage	Use a moderate amount of your blend and massage it in all over your body, or at least areas like your hands and arms, face, neck, shoulders, and if you have someone to help, your back as well. Use quicker shorter strokes if you want to perk your energy levels up, and slower longer strokes if you would prefer to encourage sleep.

Bath	Use 10-15mls of your chosen blend and add it to a warm, drawn bath. Disperse the oil with your hand, get in, and relax for about 20 minutes. Be extra careful getting into and out of the bath tub due to the oils making the surface slippery.

27. VARICOSE VEINS

Varicose veins happen when the valves in our veins become weakened and the blood begins to pool in the cavities within the veins, instead of being pushed along to the next cavity as normal. They can come about simply as a result of standing for a long time, or sitting for excessive periods. The increased weight in the pelvic region can also sometimes put pressure on the blood vessels in the pelvis and legs, causing the veins to bulge and become prominent. Poor muscle tone can also contribute to the occurrence of varicose veins. Varicose veins can also occur in the vulva (called vulval varicosities - see Haemorrhoids and Vulval Varicosities above), especially due to the extra blood flow in the pelvic area and are extremely uncomfortable especially when walking, as clothing and friction are inclined to aggravate them further.

Suggested Essential Oils for Varicose Veins	Cypress Geranium Grapefruit Lavender Lemon

Blend	Use 50ml of grapeseed carrier oil and add the following: Cypress 2 drops Geranium 2 drops Grapefruit 3 drops Lavender 2 drops Lemon 3 drops
Massage	Please note, **NEVER massage directly over the affected area of a varicose vein**, therefore, stroke the leg GENTLY upwards, avoiding direct contact with the varicosity.
Bath	Use 10-15mls of your blend and add it to a warm, drawn bath. Disperse the oil with your hand, get in, and relax for about 20 minutes. Use caution getting into and out of the bath tub as the oils will make the surface slippery.

CHAPTER 6

Your Pregnancy Skin

PREGNANCY CAN CAUSE changes in our skin – some welcome, others not so much. Pregnancy can also mean that we must address the way in which we treat some pre-existing skin conditions differently, so as not to adversely affect the baby in the womb. As I mentioned earlier, it is very important to be aware of what you are putting on your skin, but especially in pregnancy. This is because many chemical constituents and various molecules of skincare products can pass through the skin barrier, reach the bloodstream, and can also cross the placental barrier to be apparent in the baby's bloodstream and amniotic fluid.

Many women report having increased skin sensitivity in pregnancy, or experience breakouts, red patches, dry patches, or the condition called chloasma whereby a mask-like pigmentation appears on the face. Some women also experience the onset of rosacea during pregnancy, which may or may not disappear after birth.

Oh, you're glowing!

Most women are delighted with an improvement in their skin tone and texture in pregnancy, given the increase in blood flow around the body, and this is often referred to as the pregnancy 'glow'. Nonetheless, some women note the appearance of acne or pimples on their face, neck, and upper back in pregnancy and this can cause stress and concern. Such breakouts are most often due to the hormonal changes taking place in their body. Some people suggest that the gender of the baby may affect the appearance of the mother's skin, however, this may be nothing more than old wives' tales. Skin breakouts may also be a result of feeling tired and a bit run down, especially if your sleep has been broken or disturbed.

Given that your diet and your skin are inextricably linked, it is obviously important to be mindful of what you are eating when pregnant. Drinking plenty of clean water and eating lots of fresh vegetables and fruit (organic, if possible), and good quality protein will definitely benefit your skin. Light aerobic exercise and proper rest will also have a beneficial action on the skin.

It is, however, also very important to be aware of what you put ON your skin. You may find that your usual creams and lotions may react differently on your skin now that you are expecting, or that you are more sensitive to their fragrances and perhaps find them overpowering and even nauseating - even though you may have used them for years without any issue. This may require a review of your skin care routine to include products that contain ingredients to which your skin will respond more positively.

Even if your skin is not reacting strangely to your skin products of old, it is important to remember that artificial fragrances (that are found in abundance in the cosmetic industry) have been linked to hormonal disruption for both the mother and her baby. Furthermore, some ingredients used in the mainstream cosmetic industry are also carcinogenic, or lead to toxic build-up within the body. As I mentioned before, certain chemical constituents that move trans-dermally, will reach the mother's bloodstream, and subsequently, can also cross the placental blood barrier, to be present in the baby's bloodstream and also the amniotic fluid that cushions it.

Another ingredient that has no place in cosmetics, especially those that a pregnant woman will be using, is mineral oil, even though it is found in the majority of mainstream cosmetic products, and has no moisturising benefits for the skin. Yes, I know you think I must be grossly misinformed - surely I've seen all the advertisements saying how wonderfully moisturised your skin will look and feel after using certain products (that contain mineral oil)? Yes, I have. Alas, money talks, and advertising works. Mineral oil or another of its names, liquidum paraffinum, as it may appear on cosmetic labels, is a cheap by-product of the petroleum industry and it does not contain any essential fatty acids or vitamins. What it actually does is draw the skin's own moisture reserves up from the lower layers and trap it at the top of the skin so that it feels plump, and soft. However, it prevents the skin from breathing and keeps the toxins that the skin is trying to expel, within the body, leaving your organs to work harder to eliminate the toxins and waste products, via other means. It's as if the body is being covered in cling film when you apply mineral oil. Furthermore, once the product containing the mineral oil has worn off, your skin feels very dry because the moisture has been robbed from the lower layers. Therefore, you feel as if you need to apply more product, and so the cycle continues. Dry skin –– more mineral oil – depleted lower layers of skin – trapped toxins – and organs working harder to eliminate waste products.

Prolonged use of products containing mineral oil can severely deplete the skin's natural moisturising resources and may result in premature signs of ageing.

If your skin is unable to breathe and function as a method of excretion for your body, then this may put extra pressure on your digestive system and lungs as they have to pick up where the skin left off, and work harder to get rid of the body's waste products and toxins. This has a knock-on effect, and especially in pregnancy when your digestive system may have become more sluggish due to the shift in progesterone levels. There are also the physical space restrictions to consider, as your womb grows and develops which consequently results in your intestines being squashed leading to fewer, less regular or less efficient bowel movements. What this means is that your body can hold on to toxins and waste products for longer which will impact upon your energy resources and tiredness levels.

If you are experiencing breakouts due to your pregnancy, then I would suggest using essential oils that can help to balance your hormones as well as being gentle on the skin. Most essential oils show some degree of being antiseptic, so many of them will help to clear up spots and pimples. However, some are more antiseptic than others and are more relevant for skin healing and rejuvenation.

It is very important to use plant-based products that use natural oils instead of man-made mineral oil if you want your skin to be able to work at its optimum, and not to be adding to any stress or imbalance, unnecessarily. It may seem strange at first to be using oil on your face especially if you feel that your face is already producing too much oil. However, this is more than likely because you may be using products that have been stripping your skin's natural oils excessively and then it over reacts by producing even more of its natural oils. This may be due to using products that contain mineral oil and harsh cleansing agents, and in fairness, these common ingredients are hard to avoid if you're using mainstream skin products and cosmetics. The good news is; plant oils like jojoba oil are wonderful for regulating your skin's output of sebum as it has a very similar composition. After using natural, plant oils on your face for even 10 to 14 days, you will notice how well your skin looks and feels, and perhaps surprisingly, it will not feel oily or greasy.

FACIAL MASSAGE

The muscles in our jaw and face are working hard all day; they are used when we talk, when we eat, and when our face changes its expression. They are attached to our neck muscles and those covering the scalp, and when these areas become tight with tension, it also impacts the status of our face muscles. It feels good to have them worked deeply, to help remove that tension and strain. And, if we're looking at a screen for the most part of the day, we often hold our facial muscles in a tight, tense way without even realising that we haven't relaxed them in a very long time. In pregnancy, your face is still one part of your body that you can access easily - you don't have to bend, or struggle and get out of breath to reach it. By carrying out an aromatherapy facial massage at home you don't have to lie or sit on a massage couch, you can be wearing your PJs and have your hair scraped back, and you are doing wonders both for the appearance of your facial skin and for your stress levels in general.

Here's a sequence that is perfect for relaxation, and for helping to address problem areas of your skin.

After cleansing your skin, use clean fingertips and massage a moderate amount of your blended oil in small circular movements all over your face and neck. Use enough oil so that your hands and fingers can glide easily over your skin, but not so much that they slide off your skin with no friction. Do not drag your skin, especially the delicate skin around your eyes, but your cheeks and jawline will appreciate relatively deep massage using either your fingers or your knuckles. You can use wide circular movements all over your cheeks, using your knuckles and really feel the muscles react and release against your hands. It feels wonderful, and you can continue to do this for a couple of minutes to really work out the stress and tension that has built up there.

The following techniques also promote increased blood flow and oxygen to the skin, encourage lymphatic drainage and lessen damage from free-radical build-up:

- Keeping four fingers on each hand together, use their flat underside and stroke broadly across your forehead, first with one hand in one direction, and then with the other hand in the other direction.
- Using your forefingers, start at the bridge of your nose, sweep downwards along the sides of the nose, under the cheek bones, and out towards the sides of the face.
- Using the pad of your thumbs, push upwards and outwards from the innermost point of your eyebrows out towards the

outer side. Do this again, but add in a pinch between your thumb and your forefinger every centimetre or so. This may feel a little tender, but it is an excellent technique for relaxing your facial muscles.

- Tilt your chin up and using the pads of your four fingers together, glide downwards and outwards over your neck skin. This action helps to keep lymph moving towards the lymph nodes in your neck, and below your ears. Make sure that you have enough oil on your skin so that it doesn't drag.
- Finish off by using light tapotement movements, which looks like the action of playing the piano, all over your face. This feels beautiful, will invigorate the skin, and creates a fantastic vibration all over your face.

The action of the massage, combined with the therapeutic characteristics of the essential oil blend does wonders for your skin, as well as your sense of well-being. Blood flow is improved, thereby facilitating a greater supply of oxygen to the capillaries in your skin, and waste products are removed more easily. Your skin's own regenerative action is facilitated, which helps to heal spots and pimples more easily and improve the appearance and texture of the skin.

If you are doing this facial massage at night before going to bed, keep the massage actions slow and steady, to offer a more relaxing sensation.

Have a drink of cool water afterwards.

HYDROSOLS

Hydrosols, or floral waters are also beautiful to use on your skin, and even moreso in pregnancy, as they are lighter than essential oils and are beautifully refreshing. Hydrosols are a by-product of the essential oil extraction process, and they contain many of the beneficial properties of the essential oils themselves. They also have many therapeutic benefits in their own right and can be used to address skin issues like redness, broken veins, burns, or irritation. Unlike essential oils, most floral waters have the advantage of being able to be spritzed directly onto your skin or dabbed on using a cotton wool pad for them to act like a facial toner. Their fragrance will also have a beneficial action on your emotions and state of mind. Some of my favourite hydrosols are Rose Water, Lavender Water, Orange Flower Water, and Chamomile Water, but you can get many, many others. Of these four that I have mentioned, all can be used at 100%, i.e. there is no need for further dilution, except for chamomile water; it should only be used at a maximum of 10% dilution as it can have a drying effect on the skin.

If you would like to make your own blend of floral waters to create a personal floral blend, then it is a simple process of choosing your floral waters and mixing them together in a glass flask, and then storing your final product in a dark-coloured glass bottle. If you would like to use your floral water in spray form, then simply add an atomiser instead of a normal lid.

HOT CLOTH CLEANSING

Hot cloth cleansing is a gorgeous way to cleanse your skin as it is very effective at removing grime buildup and makeup. It feels beautiful on your skin and oils used make it highly nourishing. It can be carried out as follows:

Apply 5-10mls of your oil blend (detailed above) all over your face and neck. Massage into your skin, breathe deeply, and enjoy the beautiful fragrance of the essential oils in your blend. Soak a clean face flannel in a bowl or sink of warm water and wring out the excess water. Place it gently over your face, pressing lightly into your eye sockets and over your cheekbones and chin. Pat the flannel all over your face and neck and start wiping off the cleansing oil with circular movements. Rinse and repeat until the excess oil has been removed or has sunk into your skin, leaving it beautifully cleansed, refreshed, soft, and supple.

You can use this type of face cleanser on a daily basis.

Common skin conditions In pregnancy

1.   ROSACEA

Rosacea is when your skin experiences red patchy breakouts normally around the cheeks, nose, chin, and forehead, it can be more common in fair-skinned people, and also it occurs more often in women than in men. The redness can be accompanied by raised, pus-filled pimples, and in severe cases, the area around the eyes and eyelids also becomes sore, inflamed, and itchy. For some women, it accompanies their pregnancy and breastfeeding journey, and in these instances, seems to be hormonally triggered.

Aromatherapy can help to calm the inflammation and to ease the itchiness that can make rosacea so challenging to live with.

Suggested Essential Oils for Rosacea	Lavender Neroli Patchouli Roman Chamomile Rose
Soothing Face Oil for Rosacea (50ml)	Mix the following carrier oils: Rosehip oil 30ml Seabuckthorn oil 10ml Grapeseed oil 10ml Add the following essential oils: Rose 1 drop Roman chamomile 1 drop Lavender 5 drops Patchouli 1 drop Neroli 2 drops

Directions	Apply 5ml of your blend using the facial massage techniques described above.

2. ACNE

Pregnancy acne can be addressed directly by using the following blend of essential oils. This blend can be massaged into your face and left on overnight, or in hot cloth cleansing and removed after the massage. Either way, your skin will benefit from the therapeutic nature of the essential oils, and from the balancing properties of the carrier oils used.

Suggested Essential Oils for Acne	Bergamot Geranium Frankincense Lavender Rose Sweet orange
Balancing Facial Oil for Acne	Grapeseed oil 25ml Jojoba oil 10ml Rosehip oil 10ml Evening primrose oil 5ml Add the following essential oils: Bergamot 3 drops Frankincense 1 drop Geranium 2 drops Lavender 2 drops Rose 1 drop Sweet orange 2 drops
Directions:	Using clean fingertips, apply a moderate amount of your blend to acne-prone areas of your face, chest and back, and allow it to absorb into your skin.

3. CHLOASMA

Another change in facial skin that many pregnant women notice is chloasma, often called the pregnancy mask, and it occurs when darker pigmented skin develops around the forehead, cheeks, temples, and upper lip. Again, this can be as a result of the rise of pregnancy hormones in the body, this time oestrogen, which can encourage an increase in melanin production, causing the skin to look darker in some areas. Not surprisingly, sun exposure is also an important factor in the severity of the occurrence of chloasma. However, perhaps something that may not have been considered is that nutritional factors may also contribute, and it is recommended that a diet with natural sources of folates (e.g., lentils, legumes like pinto beans, avocados, broccoli, tropical fruits like mangoes, and also oranges) be consumed in pregnancy to help overcome chloasma.

What do I do about my chloasma?

Well, the good news is that for most women, their skin will return to its normal colour and tone once the baby is born, for others, it may only fade once breastfeeding comes to an end. It may be a good idea to use a daily sunblock on your face if you're prone to chloasma.

Suggested Essential Oils for Chloasma	Frankincense
	Geranium
	Lemon
	Rose

Facial Oil for Chloasma	Use the following carrier oils: Rosehip oil 20ml Apricot kernel oil 20ml Evening primrose oil 9ml Vitamin E 1 ml Add the following essential oils: Frankincense 3 drops Geranium 3 drops Lemon 3 drops Rose 1 drop

4. ECZEMA

Eczema, the condition where your skin becomes sore, itchy and sometimes weepy, usually in the creases of your elbows or behind your knees can be hereditary or linked to other inflammatory conditions like asthma. It may flare up or recede in pregnancy. If it flares up, it may be hormone related. However, stress may also be a contributing factor in your eczema getting worse.

Outside of pregnancy, it is often treated with oral or topical steroids. However, in pregnancy, these treatments are not recommended, but the good news is; there are essential oils that promote new skin growth, are pain-relieving, and anti-inflammatory that can help.

Suggested Essential Oils for Eczema	Atlas cedarwood Bergamot Frankincense Geranium Lavender Patchouli Roman chamomile Rose Vetiver

Body Oil for Eczema	Use this carrier oil base: Rosehip oil 25ml Calendula oil 10ml (Solid) Coconut oil 15ml Add the following: Atlas cedarwood 2 drops Bergamot 6 drops Rose 1 drop Or Frankincense 4 drops Lavender drops Rose 1 drop Vetiver 1 drop Or Bergamot 5 drops Geranium 2 drops Lavender 3 drops Patchouli 1 drop

Directions	The above blends can be used as a body oil and applied directly to the problematic areas, or in the bath (add 15ml to a drawn bath and relax - show extra caution getting into and out of the bath tub due to the oils making the bath surface slippery). The coconut oil content may make this blend slightly thicker to use, depending on the type of climate you live in. If it is too solid to store in a bottle, simply keep it in a glass jar or aluminium tin, and if needs be, scoop it onto your skin instead of pouring it.

5. PSORIASIS

Psoriasis is also an irritated and inflamed skin condition, but it normally appears as scaly deposits on the outer surface of the elbows, arms, and knees. It happens when your immune system is excessively responsive and causes the rate of skin production to become overly rapid, and instead of taking about a month for new skin cells to travel from the lower layers of the skin to the outside and shed, it can take as few as four or five days. This means that the skin cells at the surface do not have time to shed as well as they should, and instead they build up, forming scaly areas of skin plaque. Some people suffer considerably more with larger areas of their body being affected. Once again, pregnancy can either lessen the severity of your psoriasis, or exacerbate it, and often your normal treatment options may not work in pregnancy.

Suggested Essential Oils for Psoriasis	Bergamot Fragonia Frankincense Lavender Geranium Rose Vetiver
Body oil for Psoriasis	Calendula oil 20ml Sweet almond oil 40ml Jojoba oil 40ml Bergamot 6 drops Fragonia 5 drops Frankincense 3 drops Lavender 5 drops Geranium 3 drops Rose 1 drop Vetiver 1 drop
Directions	The above blend can be used as a body oil and applied directly to the problematic areas, or in the bath (add 15ml to a drawn bath and relax - show extra caution getting into and out of the bath tub due to the oils making the bath surface slippery).

6. STRETCH MARKS

Often before a woman even becomes pregnant, there are conversations about the dreaded 'S' word – stretch marks, and how to avoid them. From my own experience, it was one thing that I was concerned about keeping at bay during my pregnancies. Stretch marks can happen when the rate of growth of your skin has difficulty in keeping up with the rate of growth of your body underneath. Changes in skin physiology mean that structural fibres in the middle layer of your skin are stretched and often broken, causing the appearance of darker pigmented lines most often around your belly, breasts, and thighs.

Not everyone gets stretch marks, but there seem to be some factors that might make getting them more likely: stress, dehydration, rapid weight gain, and unfortunately, genetics - which like it or not, is decidedly out of our hands!

Unfortunately, stretch marks can be accompanied by tight, itchy, inflamed skin as it stretches to embrace your growing baby bump. It is not realistic to say that if you do x, y or z you will definitely not get stretch marks. However, staying hydrated, incorporating healthy oils like olive oil and coconut oil, and oils that are rich in Omega 3 like flaxseed into your diet, and keeping your skin properly nourished to improve its elasticity will help make your growing body more comfortable. From working regularly with pregnant women, in my opinion, stress is also a significant factor in how a woman's body reacts to her pregnancy, so staying relaxed, both mentally and physically and allowing your body to work properly, is very important too. Getting reflexology, going for a massage, doing yoga or going for some acupuncture are all wonderful ways of helping to stay relaxed, and physically and emotionally balanced when pregnant.

Another important thing you can do for yourself is to care for your skin and keep it properly nourished and hydrated as your pregnancy progresses. Your body diverts many of the nutrients you take in via your food to your baby, so it's important to give your skin some extra love in the form of proper moisturisation and TLC. While no cream, lotion or potion can or should say that it will 100% prevent stretch marks, improved elasticity of the skin may diminish their appearance somewhat and improve how your skin feels. Properly moisturised skin will not feel as tight or as uncomfortable, and certain beneficial ingredients may also help with inflammation and itchiness.

Suggested Essential Oils for Stretch marks	Bergamot Frankincense Geranium Lavender Neroli Rose
Body oil for Stretch Marks	Rosehip oil 27ml Thistle oil 35ml Sweet almond oil 35ml Vit. E 2ml Bergamot 6 drops Frankincense 6 drops Geranium 4 drops Lavender 5 drops Neroli 2 drop Rose 1 drop Apply to your bump, thighs, and breasts twice a day. Can be applied to dry or damp skin. This blend can also be used in the bath: Add 10-15ml to an already drawn, warm bath, and relax. As always, be extra careful getting into and out of the bath tub because the oils will make the surface slippery.

Chapter 7

Labour and Post-Partum

THE THOUGHT OF labour and birth can bring about mixed emotions in a woman, and often her partner too. Some people like to opt for the sticking their head in the sand approach, but I am very much an advocate of being fully informed about what can happen, and what our bodies are perfectly designed, and wonderfully able to do. Unfortunately, in many instances, birth has turned into an overly medical event and we are subjected to less than supportive or encouraging reports of not very pleasant experiences, that may leave a woman both physically and mentally scarred, and ultimately, fearful of the situation.

It doesn't have to be this way, and I would like to promote the idea of labour and birth being a very positive and special time for a woman and her partner, and of course for the baby being born. Let it be a calm time, one that is nurturing and respectful of the natural and wonderful process that is birth, and one that can be enjoyed and remembered as a beautiful time in your life. I have enjoyed three very positive birthing experiences, and I would like you to be able to enjoy your best birth too.

In terms of aromatherapy, it can help throughout the labour process in so many ways. Think about the emotions that you want to promote, and those which you would like to lessen. Reflect on how we want to support the body physically and mentally so that it can carry out its amazing birthing actions as intended.

Positives to Promote in Labour	Negatives to Reduce in Labour
Calmness	Anxiety
Confidence	Discomfort
Connection	Disempowerment
Delight	Exhaustion
Enjoyment	Fear
Euphoria	Lack of confidence
Excitement	Loss of control
Happiness	Mistrust
Joy	Nervousness
Love	Pain
Power	Panic
Quietness	Sickness
Reassurance	
Relaxation	
Respect	
Strength	
Wisdom	

By creating an environment whereby the positive list above is facilitated, then you are giving yourself the best possible chance at a positive birthing experience - even if everything doesn't go exactly as planned. However, you will feel assured that you have given yourself every opportunity for your birthing experience to be as positive as possible, allowing your body and mind to operate in a way that is supportive of the natural birthing experience.

LABOUR

I know that it's difficult to keep excitement at bay knowing that you're going to be meeting your baby relatively soon, so in early stages of labour, if your waters, or membranes, have yet to release, you may really find the benefits of a warm bath to help keep you calm and relaxed. Your body may be experiencing period-like cramping or mild surging in your lower back and abdomen, however this may be irregular and not following any true pattern. If it's not proper labour, then a bath may allow the cramping to subside, but if labour is actually happening, then the surges or cramping will remain, albeit in a more comfortable fashion.

Suggested Essential Oils for Early Labour	Clary sage Frankincense Lavender Rosewood Sandalwood Ylang ylang
Blend	Use 50ml of carrier oil (e.g. Sweet almond oil, or grapeseed oil) Add the following essential oils: Clary Sage 1 drop Frankincense 3 drops Lavender 4 drops Rosewood 2 drops Sandalwood 2 drops Ylang ylang 1 drop
Directions	Use 10-15ml of the blend dispersed through a warm bath. This blend can also be used for massage if you feel that you would like to have your back, sacrum, buttocks or thighs rubbed, or have pressure applied.

Remember, early labour for some women can last many hours, and may even run into days, so it is important to eat, rest when you can, or even better, sleep, and stay properly hydrated.

For labour to progress, we really want to be encouraging the proper flow of hormones, and anything that is conducive to the release of oxytocin. We want to inhibit the release of adrenaline as it is counter-productive to the effects of oxytocin, so essential oils that promote calmness and relaxation are important, as are ones that are muscle relaxants, and that encourage deep breathing and focus.

Sometimes in labour, you may find yourself not wanting to be touched, thereby ruling out massage; you may also not want to be in the bath, instead preferring to be mobile and walking around, so ruling out bath oils. This is when your oil burner or plug-in diffuser will prove a great alternative.

To stay calm	Frankincense 1 drop
	Geranium 1 drop
	Lavender 1 drop
To alleviate nausea	Peppermint 1 drop
	Lemon 2 drops

In an acute situation, inhalation of essential oils from a tissue works very well:

To regulate rapid or shallow breathing	Use the following on a tissue and breathe in directly:
	Atlas cedarwood 1 drop
	Frankincense 1 drop
	Sandalwood 1 drop

If you are experiencing painful surges (contractions), applying pressure to the sacrum or hips can be very helpful.

50ml carrier oil of your choice
Lavender 4 drops
Frankincense 2 drops
Roman chamomile 2 drops
Vetiver 1 drop
Rose otto 1 drop
Clary sage 1 drop

Sometimes in labour your lips can become very dry, and your nose blocked or stuffed up (perhaps only on one side) - I recommend using a (non-petroleum based) peppermint lip balm as this addresses both the issue of dry lips, and the peppermint essential oil helps to open up your nasal passages, making breathing easier. This can also help if you are feeling nauseous in labour, as the peppermint essential oil can help lift the queasy sensation.

It is also quite common to feel very hot in labour, and a facial spritz is a quick and easy way to help you to cool down. I can recommend the use of hydrosols such as rose or lavender floral waters; they will feel good on your skin, and their fragrances will be uplifting and refreshing. You can spray the lavender or rose hydrosol liberally over your face and chest to help cool you down and keep your skin feeling moist and hydrated. If you would like to enjoy only the benefits of their fragrance, simply mist them into the air about you.

BIRTHING

As baby is crowning, it can be helpful to use a warm compress against your perineum. It will help the skin to stretch more easily around the baby's emerging head, lessening the chance of perineal tearing.

Add a tablespoon of sweet almond oil to a bowl of warm water and soak a flannel in it. Wring out the flannel and apply it directly to the perineum. Continue doing this for as long as this feels comfortable until the baby is born.

There is no need to use essential oils here as it is too close to baby's emerging face.

POST-PARTUM

After the baby is born, a woman's body seems to survive on happy hormones for a while, and we often feel like we are Superwoman (which we are!), and that we could easily run a marathon. We are so delighted with our new baby and spend most of our time just looking at them and holding them and kissing them - wrapped up in the euphoria of newborn love.

However, after having given birth, you may have vaginal bruising, pelvic floor tears, and stitches, or haemorrhoids to contend with, and if you have given birth by C-section, your wound will also be painful and bruised as it recovers from the surgery. Then, the pregnancy and birth hormones start to subside, and we experience what are commonly known as the baby blues. This tends to happen about two or three days after the baby's arrival and can last from a few days to a couple of weeks. These feelings can coincide with the feeling of exhaustion from having survived on very little sleep over the previous few days, or being overwhelmed as the realisation of your new responsibility sinks in. You may feel extremely tearful and emotional, without really understanding why. This is all very normal and nothing to get too concerned about (I know it all feels a bit overwhelming when you're in it, and I do not mean to be dismissive of it in any way). However, having helpful, supportive, and positive people around you who will help with the practicalities of life with a new-born is extremely important. They will be able to do the everyday household stuff like making meals, doing laundry, and perhaps looking after other children, thereby allowing you to rest and spend time with your new baby. With this help and support, these tearful days, and feeling of overwhelm pass.

However, if you experience prolonged periods of feeling like you're not able to cope, and think that it may be more like post natal depression, please do not feel you must hide your feelings or pretend that everything is ok. Please make sure to tell your public health nurse, GP or a close confidante, so that you can get proper help and support.

POST PARTUM SORE/TENDER BITS

Suggested Essential Oils to ease Post-Partum Sore/Tender Bits	Frankincense
	Geranium
	Lavender
	Roman chamomile
	Rosewood
	Vetiver

Blend	Use 50ml of sweet almond oil and add the following: Frankincense 2 drops Geranium 2 drops Lavender 3 drops Roman chamomile 2 drops Rosewood 2 drops Vetiver 1 drop
Bath	Use 10-15mls of your chosen blend and add it to a warm, drawn bath. Disperse the oil with your hand, get in, and relax for about 20 minutes. Remember to be extra careful getting into and out of the bath tub as the oils can make the surface extremely slippery. Furthermore, your legs may feel a little wobbly for a few days after the birth, so it's important for a loved one to be there to help you.
Sitz Bath	If you don't feel like getting into a full bath, a Sitz bath is perfect to help ease vaginal or perineal bruising. Add 10ml of your blend to a Sitz bath filled with warm water and disperse it through the water. Rest your bottom in it and relax for about 10 minutes. Pat the area dry with a clean towel.

POST-PARTUM HAEMORRHOIDS

Sometimes haemorrhoids appear as a result of strained pushing in labour. Please refer back to Chapter 5 for how to treat them.

BREASTS AND BREASTFEEDING

Your breasts will be experiencing dramatic changes too as your milk comes in to replace the initial colostrum, and it's important to look after them, attending to any discomfort straight away so as not to let the situation worsen. Some women have little to no trouble when nursing their baby, but for others, it may take a while to get comfortable with breastfeeding, and to establish a good latch position for baby to feed. Please do be patient as it will be really worthwhile and rewarding when breastfeeding is established and comfortable. Hiring the support of a lactation consultant is money very well spent, even if it is not your first time breastfeeding, as each baby is different and may require their latch to be checked. Studies have shown that women enjoy a longer, more positive breastfeeding journey if they have the right support in establishing it properly at the start.

In the case of painful breasts or nipples, here are some blends that may prove helpful. However, bearing in mind that your baby will be much more sensitive to the likes of essential oils, we are using the lower dilution of 0.25%, compared to the 1% dilution that we have previously been working with.

A good idea is to apply the oils after an episode of breastfeeding, although, I do realise that this may be challenging as your new-born will most likely feed very regularly. Nonetheless, please make sure to remove the excess oil from your breasts and nipples before having your baby close to your skin, or when breastfeeding.

SORE/CRACKED NIPPLES

When breastfeeding, your nipples can become very sore and cracked if your baby's latch is in any way incorrect. Sometimes, the baby will not open his or her mouth wide enough to grasp the breast and nipple properly, at times only sucking on your nipple, and this creates a lipstick-like shape, which can be extremely painful. It is important to get baby's latch right from the start if breastfeeding is to be comfortable.

Suggested Essential Oils for Sore/ Cracked Nipples	Lavender Roman chamomile
Blend	Melt 25ml coconut oil (solid) in a bain marie so that it turns to liquid. As it is cooling and beginning to solidify slightly again, add 25ml calendula oil, and then the following essential oils, and stir well: Lavender 2 drops Roman chamomile 2 drops Store in a dark-coloured jar.
Topical application	Apply a small amount to each sore/cracked nipple after breastfeeding. Remove any excess before your baby re-latches.

BREAST ENGORGEMENT

When your milk comes in properly, normally a couple of days after your baby is born, it can lead to your breasts becoming engorged. This means that your breasts can feel stretched, hot, hard, and very sensitive. A cool compress can offer some welcome relief.

Suggested Essential Oils for Breast Engorgement	Geranium Lavender Mandarin Roman chamomile

Blend	Grapeseed oil 50ml Geranium 1 drop Lavender 1 drop Mandarin 1 drop Roman chamomile 1 drop
Compress	Add 10ml of your blend to a bowl/basin of cool water and mix it through with your hand. Soak a face flannel in the oil/water, wring out, and then apply directly to the breasts. Leave on for about 5 minutes on each breast. Rinse and repeat. You can do one breast at a time, or have two flannels and use one on both breasts at the same time. It may help to be in a semi-reclined or seated position so that you can relax with the compress applied. Wipe any trace of your oil blend away before baby re-latches for breastfeeding.

MASTITIS

Mastitis occurs when your breast tissue becomes inflamed, perhaps as a result of a milk duct that has not cleared, or of an infection that has entered your breast tissue through a damaged nipple. It is extremely painful and can be accompanied by fever, and flu-like symptoms, making you feel very unwell. It is important to contact your GP, public health nurse or midwife in case you require antibiotics. Essential oils can help with the inflammation and potentially the infection.

Suggested Essential Oils for Mastitis	Fragonia Lavender Roman chamomile Rose
Blend	Use 50ml of Grapeseed oil and add the following: Fragonia 1 drop Lavender 1 drop Roman chamomile 1 drop Rose 1 drop
Compress	Add 10mls of your blend to a bowl/basin of cool water and mix it through with your hand. Soak a face flannel in the oil/water, wring out, and then apply directly to the breasts. Leave on for about 5 minutes on each breast. Rinse and repeat. You can do one breast at a time, or have two flannels and use them on both breasts at the same time. It may help to be in a semi-reclined or seated position so that you can relax with the compress applied. Wipe any trace of your oil blend away before baby re-latches for breastfeeding.

BLOCKED MILK DUCT

Generally, the best way to unblock a milk duct is to have your baby feed as often as possible. With regular feeding, the blockage can clear and you will suddenly notice that the pain subsides, and the tenderness begins to alleviate. However, using a compress and/or massage can also help.

Suggested Essential Oils for Blocked Milk Ducts	Geranium Lemon Patchouli
Blend	50ml Grapeseed oil Geranium 1 drop Lemon 2 drops Patchouli 1 drop
Compress	Add 10mls of your blend to a bowl/basin of warm water and mix it through with your hand. Soak a face flannel in the oil/water, wring out, and then apply directly to the breasts. Leave on for about 5 minutes on each breast. Rinse and repeat. You can do one breast at a time, or have two flannels and use them on both breasts at the same time. It may help to be in a semi-reclined or seated position so that you can relax with the compress applied. Wipe any trace of your oil blend away before baby re-latches for breastfeeding.

Massage	Using a moderate amount of your blend, massage each breast all over. Try and use your knuckles to go deeper into the breast tissue. Proceed very slowly as this will more than likely be extremely tender. Continue this for a few minutes on each breast. You can do this 4 times a day until the blocked duct clears. Wipe any trace of your oil blend away before baby re-latches for breastfeeding.

Glossary

Antiseptic	Prevents the growth of disease-causing organisms
Antimicrobial	Reduces the growth of microbes
Antispasmodic	Relaxes smooth muscle (e.g. muscles of the digestive tract or uterus)
Antiviral	Prevents the growth or spread of a virus
Aphrodisiac	Heightens or encourages a person's sexual response
Astringent	Causes the tightening or constriction of skin cells
Carminative	Reduces flatulence
Cytophylactic	Encourages skin healing
Deodorising	Reduces bad odours
Digestive	Aids proper digestion
Diuretic	Causes increased flow of urine for the removal of waste products
Emmenagogue	Encourages or stimulates menstrual flow
Euphoric	Promotes mental highs
Expectorant	Encourages the production and expulsion of phlegm
Hormone Regulator	Balances hormones

Immune stimulant	Promotes better functioning of your immune system
Meditative	Encourages a relaxed, calm and clear-minded state
Oestrogenic	Has an oestrogen-like action or effect on the body
Sedative	Promotes calmness or sleepiness
Soporific	Induces tiredness and sleepiness
Stimulant	Encourages a more alert response
TCS (Topical Circulatory Stimulant)	Improves blood flow to a specific area by being applied to the skin
Vasoconstrictor	Reduces the size of a vein or capillary to restrict blood flow in that area.
Vulnerary	Useful in the healing of wounds

Bibliography

Essential Oil Safety 2nd ed, Tisserand and Young, 2013

Essential Oil Safety, Tisserand and Balacs, 1991

Principles of Anatomy and Physiology 9th ed., Tortora/Grabowski, 2000

The Complete Guide to Aromatherapy, Battaglia, 1997

Unreasonable Risk – How to avoid cancer from Cosmetics and Personal Care Products", Samuel S. Epstein, M.D., 2001

Useful Resources

BUYING ESSENTIAL OILS, CARRIER OILS, AND CONTAINERS

Company (Ireland)	Essential Oils	Carrier Oils	Containers
Atlantic Aromatics www.atlanticaromatics. com	✓	✓	
Bomar www.bomar.ie	✓	✓	✓
Ogam www.ogamoils.ie	✓	✓	

Company (UK)	Essential Oils	Carrier Oils	Containers
Tisserand www.tisserand.com	✓	✓	
Aromantic www.aromantic.co.uk	✓	✓	✓
Naturally Thinking www.naturallythinking. com	✓	✓	✓
Quinessence www.quinessence.com	✓	✓	✓

FURTHER AROMATHERAPY READING:

Aromatherapy – An A-Z by Patricia Davis, ISBN: 0-85207-295-3

Aromatherapy in Midwifery Practice by Denise Tiran, ISBN: 0-7020-1978-X

Aromatherapy for a Healthy Lifestyle by Shirley Price, ISBN:1-902328-33-7

The Art of Aromatherapy by Robert Tisserand, ISBN: 0-85207-140-X

The Fragrant Mind by Valerie Ann Worwood, ISBN: 0-535-40799-6

FURTHER POSITIVE PREGNANCY READING AND RESOURCES:

Birth and Breastfeeding by Michel Odent, ISBN: 978-1905570065

Childbirth without Fear by Grantly Dick-Read and Michel Odent, ISBN: 978-1780660554

Ina May's Guide to Childbirth by Ina May Gaskin, ISBN: 978-0553381153

Spiritual Midwifery by Ina May Gaskin, ISBN: 978-1570671043

The Better Birth Book by Tracy Donegan, ISBN: 978-1904148876

The New Pregnancy and Childbirth by Sheila Kitzinger, ISBN: 0-14-026353-5

Gentlebirth – Brain Training App for Birth (Affiliate Link)

http://www.gentlebirth.com/ambassadors/idevaffiliate.php?id=160

Final note from the author

I hope that you enjoy reading this book and that you find the information contained herein useful. If you have any questions related to aromatherapy in pregnancy, or would like to share your pregnancy aromatherapy experiences, please feel free to join our Facebook support group – "AromaBump – Aromatherapy in Pregnancy", we'd love to see you there!

- Please also remember to check out the extra video bonuses – you can find them at www.AromaBump.com
- You can also connect with me on Facebook, Twitter and Instagram @AromaBump
- If you would like to get in touch directly, you can do so at lisa@ lisaheeney.com

Wishing you a wonderful pregnancy and birthing experience!

Lisa Heeney

Index

Lightning Source UK Ltd.
Milton Keynes UK
UKOW02f1806191116
288062UK00001B/3/P

9 781524 662639